M000200886

THE ICE SCULPTURE DIET

THE
ICE
SCULPTURE
DIET

THE COMPLETE GUIDE TO
Freeze Fat & Find a New You

ANTHONY D. GALLO

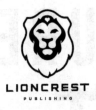

LIONCREST
PUBLISHING

COPYRIGHT © 2021 ANTHONY D. GALLO

All rights reserved.

THE ICE SCULPTURE DIET

The Complete Guide to Freeze Fat & Find a New You

ISBN   978-1-5445-1867-1 *Hardcover*

978-1-5445-1866-4 *Paperback*

978-1-5445-1865-7 *Ebook*

CONTENTS

CONTENTS

ACKNOWLEDGMENTS

Writing a book is harder than I thought but also more rewarding than I imagined. I want to thank my wife, Amy, for putting up with the crazy book publishing process over the last twelve months. Early on, when I had the idea to write *The Ice Sculpture Diet*, you pushed me to finish the manuscript. Without you, this may have stayed an idea in my head.

I also want to thank my mother, father, and sisters, Melissa and Cristina, for dealing with the unusual diet, exercise, and biohacking experiments I tried while growing up. The ability to explore and be curious without being criticized is what helped me discover this plan.

Finally, I want to thank my coworkers at Audible. Working for Audible has been an amazing experience, and seeing authors and creators share their work inspired me to share my own. PS: thanks for all the audiobooks!

INTRODUCTION

THE JOURNEY BEGINS

A friend was drunk and in tears. "I'm too over-weight for anyone to love me," he shouted, loud enough to be heard over the party music.

I saw the pain he was feeling. I had been there. I turned to him and said, "You can change anything about yourself if you change the way you think about yourself." While the words were intended for him, I knew they were for me too.

I looked down. I was overweight myself. How could I give a friend advice if I wasn't practicing what I preached? I looked around at the people chugging vodka sodas and dancing. It all clicked together in a second of understanding. In that moment, I was ready for a change.

I woke up the next morning with a mild hangover, but something was different. I had an unfamiliar energy coursing through my body. In the months that followed that night, I lost more than 35 pounds with a motivation I had never experienced before.

The weight loss changed my body. It also changed what I thought was possible.

Most importantly, I had a different mindset about weight loss. I had a vision guiding me toward my goals and a new appreciation for beliefs. I gained some weight, and I lost some more weight. I read weight loss studies and tried out their techniques. Some techniques worked, and others did not. The book you're holding now is a collection of everything that worked for me along the way.

THE STARTING POINT

If you're reading this, then chances are you're trying to reach your ideal weight. Maybe you've struggled with weight loss. Maybe, like me, you've stood in the mirror pinching your belly fat, wondering, *How the hell can I make this go away?*

I've been there. I was bullied as a child for being overweight. Even after losing weight and seeing what was possible, I still had doubts, and I still had weight to lose.

I suffered through diets, not eating enough, and feeling weak throughout the day. I had stubborn fat that seemed like it would never disappear. I watched my weight bounce up and down on the scale without a clue as to why.

Losing 35 pounds was a step in the right direction, but I wouldn't discover how to truly lose stubborn fat until years later, while stuck at home during the COVID-19 lockdown.

I discovered a new technique after doing deep research. I combined a few things to make it all work holistically. Once I found the keys that worked, I created a plan of action. I packaged everything into a series of parts and steps—a plan that kept me feeling satisfied with the food I ate and allowed me to lose fat and gain muscle. Most importantly, the plan was simple, so I could stick to it.

After following the plan for six months, I saw my abs again.

That plan is outlined in the chapters to follow. I call it the Ice Sculpture Diet.

In this book, I'll show you how to lose weight easily in three parts. In *The Foundation*, we'll learn the science of weight loss and tools to make it easy. In *The Freeze*, we'll focus on a clear method for targeted fat reduction to break through plateaus. Finally, in *Mindset and Muscle*, we'll look at developing a routine and maintaining the mindset necessary to power through the obstacles ahead.

You'll learn the basics of how the body works so that you can adjust based on your body's needs. You'll learn how to use the latest in technology to make tracking progress easy. You'll gain everything you need to break through old plateaus using fat freezing methods. Finally, you'll know how to readjust your beliefs so that you can make progress beyond what you believe is possible today.

WHO AM I?

My name is Anthony D. Gallo. I'm a certified personal trainer, life-long nutrition enthusiast, and a biohacker at heart. I'm also Director of Product Analytics for Audible.com, so you know we're going to have some fun tracking data throughout this book.

This book isn't a magic pill, though. It's a set of researched, refined steps to help you lose weight and love the way you look. Does it work? Yes. I've followed it and seen it work firsthand, even when all of my state's gyms were closed down for COVID-19. For this diet, you won't need to visit a gym if you don't want to, but you will need to take action.

As you continue to read, I'll ask you to let down your guard for a little bit, allowing yourself to experiment with the ideas I outline. Some of these ideas are new, and some of them are distilled to make the *Ice Sculpture Diet* work better for you.

If you follow the steps I outline, you will not only lose weight, but you will also learn a great deal about yourself. In some ways, what you learn about yourself may be more valuable than the weight loss you experience.

If all that sounds good to you now and you are ready to open your mind, prepare yourself for change, and start losing weight. Let's begin *The Foundation*.

PART I

THE FOUNDATION

PART I

THE
FOUNDATION

CHAPTER 1

WHY TRADITIONAL DIETS AND EXERCISE ONLY GET YOU SO FAR

We all have that one friend. You know, the guy or gal who's always trying out a new diet or exercise plan. They've had some success here and there. Maybe they lost a few pounds, only to regain the weight a few months later. I have something to admit. That person was me before I learned what I am going to teach you here.

There are many reasons why people struggle with traditional diet and exercise plans. In this chapter,

I'll walk you through the common issues I see and how to solve them. We'll start first with the problems surrounding popular restrictive diets.

TRADITIONAL FOOD-SPECIFIC RESTRICTION DIETS

Popular diets tend to require you to eat only certain types of food. Some examples include keto, paleo, grain-free, vegetarian, and carnivore diets.

If you follow these plans, there's a chance you'll lose weight. Some are very effective—for a short period of time. But two or three years down the line, people on these plans often gain back all the weight they lost.

MY KETO DIET JOURNEY

I was a huge fan of keto for a period of time. I lost a lot of weight and felt excellent while I was on it. So, why didn't I stick to it forever? Here are two reasons:

1. I started losing my hair
2. I couldn't eat the foods I enjoyed, like rice

When I was starting keto, it was tough to find articles saying anything bad about it or that it could potentially lead to hair loss. A few Reddit deep dives later, I discovered that very low carb diets could have a negative impact on hormones. Between hormone changes and the fact that I was missing key vitamins in my diet, I lost some hair.

These kinds of details about diets are hard to find online, particularly with diets that have a cult-like following. People only promote their positive experiences. These amplified stories get a lot of attention, and the negative experiences are attributed to other factors or drowned out in the noise.

I don't say this to scare you away from low-carb diets completely. I still recommend them as a great short-term way to lose weight. That said, these diets aren't long-term solutions for most people. I developed the *Ice Sculpture Diet* so that you can stick with it for the long term.

WHY FOOD-RESTRICTION DIETS ARE HARD

We're bombarded with temptations all day long. Whether it's having dinner and drinks with friends or wanting to try something new at Costco, the temptations make it difficult to stick to a diet that restricts us from eating specific foods.

As you'll discover soon, I recommend eating whatever foods fit within your macronutrient levels. We'll talk more about how to figure out what your nutrient levels are. We'll also talk about how to make sure you're eating with your health in mind.

INTENSE EXERCISE PLANS—THE GOOD AND THE BAD

You probably also have that friend who is always sweating hard at Barry's Boot Camp or an Equinox Training. Like traditional diets, these exercise programs can work—for a time.

Sure, I know some people who stick to these plans and show up every week. I also know a lot of people who try these for a month and burn out, never to return again.

WHY ARE INTENSE EXERCISE PLANS SO HARD TO STICK TO?

It's common to get excited when you start making

changes in your life. Your body releases positive brain chemicals when you do an intense workout for the first time. The problem here is that it's easy to jump headfirst into the deep end before you're ready. You might end up going all-in for a few weeks, only to run out of gas.

Your body needs time to adapt. If you go in with 100 percent effort for a few weeks after not exercising at all, your body is going to tell you to stop. It won't speak to you with words, but it will speak to you with pain.

The truth is, you burn more calories while you sleep than you burn in an intense workout. Don't believe me? When we calculate your personal calorie burn rate in Chapter 2, you will see this for yourself.

Throughout this book, I'll suggest simple movements to get you to your target weight goals. There are benefits to exercising. Working out while dieting will allow you to eat a little bit more. There are also definite, well-studied benefits to strength-training and cardio exercise. However, our focus for this book will be on weight loss. To support you after you hit your goal, I will touch on the keys to building muscle in a bonus chapter at the end of the book.

ROADBLOCKS: GETTING PAST YOUR WEIGHT LOSS PLATEAUS

Anyone who has achieved some level of weight loss has been here before—the land of plateaus. I've seen many people progress through their weight loss journey, only to hit this roadblock. When they check the scale each morning, they don't see a change for days or weeks on end. Worse, their weight goes up on some days. The whole process is confusing and frustrating.

The land of plateaus often causes the best of us to quit. The good news is that I have a solution. In Part II, I'll show you how to break past plateaus using fat freezing. This freezing process was the key that helped me pass through all the plateaus I faced. After adding this to my routine, I knew that even if the scale wasn't moving, I was losing fat. We'll also talk about limiting beliefs and how to overcome them in Part III of the book.

So, rest assured: you don't always have to trust the

scale. Some days it will be up, and some days it will be down, especially if you weigh yourself at different times throughout the day. By following the steps I outline, you will see dramatic changes not only on the scale but in the mirror too.

Keep this in mind as we progress.

Now that we've talked about why most diet and exercise routines don't work, it's time to discover a better way for weight loss using a simple formula. Turn the page now to learn how to calculate exactly what your body needs to start losing weight.

CHAPTER 2

GETTING STARTED

TRACKING CALORIE BURN RATE

Fat reduction is a science. Once you understand the basic calculations, you'll be equipped with everything you need to succeed.

As I mentioned in the last chapter, we're going to follow an *eat any type of food* approach. You can eat anything as long as it fits within your body's calorie threshold. You can easily manage calories and log the foods you eat with some apps that we'll talk about soon. Tracking will be vital to your success, and it's a lot easier than it sounds. When you're able to compare calories logged against calories burned, you can guarantee at least some level of weight loss.

Every chapter in this book builds on previous chapters. We'll start here with a solid understanding of your body's needs so we can build the proper foundation. We'll then grow from there, adding in fat freezing and mindset changes, so you can reach your ideal weight with ease.

THE BASAL METABOLIC RATE

Everyone's body burns a minimum amount of calories throughout the day to maintain life-sustaining functions, like breathing and brain activity. You burn calories even when you're asleep. But how many calories do you burn? What are the factors that affect that number? To answer these questions, you'll need to calculate your Basal Metabolic Rate (BMR).

Your BMR is the estimated number of calories that a person of your height, weight, age, and gender burns over twenty-four hours. Knowing your BMR allows you to understand how many calories you'll burn in a day even if you didn't exercise. Note that your BMR estimate can differ from your actual burn rate if you have more muscle mass than the average person.

For example, a bodybuilder with 10 to 20 pounds more muscle mass than an average person has a higher actual burn rate than their BMR estimates. This is because muscle mass burns more calories than regular body mass.

We're going to work with BMR throughout this book, so let's calculate yours now.

HOW TO CALCULATE YOUR BMR

You can find various formulas for BMR online, but I use the ones below (known as the Harris-Benedict equation):

Men: 66 + (6.23 x Weight in Pounds) + (12.7 x Height in Inches) - (6.8 x Age in Years)

Women: 655 + (4.35 x Weight in Pounds) + (4.7 x Height in Inches) - (4.7 x Age in Years)

To understand this in practice, let's calculate my current BMR. I'm a male who is 155 pounds, 71 inches tall, and thirty years old.

Here's the math using the formula above:

$$66 + (6.23 \times 155) + (12.7 \times 71) - (6.8 \times 30) = \mathbf{1{,}729.35}$$
calories a day

So, my BMR number is roughly 1,729 calories a day. Knowing this, I can assume that if I ate exactly 1,729 calories a day and did no exercise, I wouldn't gain or lose any weight.

Now it's your turn. Calculate your BMR and burn that number into your mind for the next few weeks and months. Remembering your BMR will help you make progress, so write it down.

Once you calculate your BMR, losing weight becomes a lot clearer. You can use it to calculate how much weight you will lose in a single day. You can even use it to calculate a daily calorie maximum intake if you want to lose a specific number of pounds by a certain date.

Many people pay personal trainers for an initial session just to understand their BMR. Now that you know how to do this for yourself, you can skip that session.

USE WHAT THE BMR CALCULATION TELLS YOU

While we will add calories to our BMR number later for exercise, it is easy to assume that you burn more calories than what the BMR equation tells you.

Don't be tempted to add extra calories to your burn rate. If you want to lose weight, the first step is to accept the baseline numbers so that you can build off them. While starting off, use the BMR equation above and work with the number you get. We can be a little bit more flexible later once the weight starts coming off.

SO, YOU CALCULATED YOUR BMR. NOW WHAT?

Knowing that I burn at least 1,729 calories a day, I can calculate how much food I have to eat to lose weight. I can also calculate almost exactly how long it will take to lose 5, 10, or 15 pounds based on my "intake number," or the number of calories I'm consuming each day.

Before we get into calculating how long it will take to lose weight, let's first talk about food tracking. Food tracking is going to be critical for you to see success in your weight-reduction plan, so pay attention. I'll go into more detail on technology for tracking this in Chapter 3. For now, it's worth mentioning some simple ways to track food because of how important this is for your foundational weight loss.

FOOD TRACKING MADE EASY USING YOUR SMARTPHONE

Back in the '80s and '90s, dieters tracked their food intake by writing it down in a little notebook. It's no wonder most people thought of tracking as a chore. Back then, it was difficult to figure out the calories in common foods. Smartphone apps have made that process much simpler. After a few days of tracking things, you'll notice it will become part of a routine.

There are two free apps I recommend for food tracking: Fitbit or MyFitnessPal (MFP). Both are available on iOS and Android. I recommend downloading one of these while you're reading this page.

I personally use Fitbit's app. I'll admit I switched over to Fitbit after Under Armour bought MyFitnessPal back in 2015. Ever since that acquisition, the MyFitnessPal app has a lot more ads, which I find intrusive to the logging experience. That said, MyFitnessPal's food database is much larger than Fitbit's, so it is easier to find less common foods through MFP. I suggest testing both apps and picking the one that you find easiest to use. The more comfortable you are with the app experience, the easier it will be to log.

In the next chapter, I outline how I use Fitbit's app to sync my steps and weight as well. This keeps both calories consumed and calories burned visible within a single app. Having both numbers tracked in a single app, along with weight, makes the whole routine very easy to maintain.

If you think tracking might be difficult, both MyFitnessPal and Fitbit also have a barcode scanning feature. With the scanning option, you can scan a food's barcode so that you don't have to search for the foods you're eating. I use this feature all the time to make food logging faster and simpler.

BE HONEST

The goal of food tracking is to be as honest as possible. If you're eating a plate of rice and there's no barcode to scan, you have to use your best judgment when logging portion sizes.

I tend to purposely overcount so that I don't go in the wrong direction. It's easy to underestimate how many calories you eat. If you underestimate, you'll be scratching your head, wondering why you aren't losing weight after a few weeks.

I had some trouble with measuring portion sizes when I first started logging food. How many ounces was that flank steak I just ate? Do I have to log the dressing on my salad too? How many tablespoons of Caesar was on that salad? Things get a lot easier after you start tracking. You learn how many calories are in common foods and can estimate them more easily.

A cheap food scale is also helpful when you start tracking. For me, using a food scale removed the mystery surrounding portions, making it easier to accurately measure what I was eating.

With your BMR in hand, your food-tracking app installed, and your commitment to keeping an honest food log, you're ready to start calculating how long it will take to lose weight.

LOSE ONE POUND A WEEK USING BMR AND FOOD TRACKING

You can use simple math to figure out how to lose a pound (or more) of fat.

Use the formula below to calculate how many days it would take to lose 1 pound. Keep in mind that 1 pound of fat equals roughly 3,500 calories.

$$\frac{3{,}500}{-1 \times (\textit{Daily calories burned} - \textit{Daily Calories Eaten})}$$

In other words, to figure out how many days it would take to lose 1 pound of fat, just divide the 3,500 calories by the calorie deficit you're achieving every day.

HYPOTHETICAL EXAMPLES

For the examples below, I will use my BMR, which is about 1,700.

Example 1: Eat 1,700 calories a day and burn 1,700 calories a day.

Net Calories: 0.

Days to Lose 1 lb. of Fat: Forever (I'm not gaining or losing anything!).

Example 2: I eat 1,500 calories a day and burn 1,700 calories.

Net Calories: -200 calories.

Days to Lose 1 lb. of Fat: 17.5 days (3,500/200)

Seventeen and a half days is not too bad, considering we haven't added in extra calories burned from exercise or movement yet. Your BMR number is just the calories you burn by being alive. Simple exercise, like walking, will allow you to eat more.

HOW TO EAT MORE AND LOSE WEIGHT

I usually eat right at my BMR of 1,729 calories per day, but I mainly use light exercise (walking) to maintain a caloric deficit every day. I recommend you add light exercise to your plan as well.

Whatever calories you burn during exercise can be added to your BMR in the formulas above. With a quick search online, you can easily find out calories burned during common cardio exercises. Like with food tracking, the key is to be as honest as possible, so you see results.

As I said earlier, you don't have to exercise as part of the *Ice Sculpture Diet* if you don't want to. You can maintain a caloric deficit and use the fat freezing techniques we'll discuss later. These two factors alone will help you reduce fat. That said, you can easily increase your burn rate by adding walking to your routine. I recommend walking ten thousand steps a day. This is a relatively attainable goal once you start walking daily. Walking is great for you, low impact, and easy enough to do regularly.

HOW MANY CALORIES ARE BURNED IN 10,000 STEPS?

Ten thousand steps is roughly five miles of walking, with minor variance depending on your stride length. General studies have shown that one mile of walking can burn between 65 to 100 calories. So, if you walk ten thousand steps a day, you can safely estimate that you're burning between 325 to 500 calories extra on top of your BMR.

If I combine ten thousand steps with my personal BMR of 1,700, then my new daily-calories burned number is 2,200. See how below and try filling in these numbers for yourself.

Here's the math:

> **Calories Burned:** 1,700 BMR calories burned + 500 calories (10,000 steps = roughly 500 calories burned for my size) = 2,200 calories.

> **Calories Eaten:** 1,700 consumed.

> **Net Calories:** -500 calories.

At a caloric deficit of 500 calories, I should lose a pound in about seven days. This is a safe weight loss rate for most people, but be sure to discuss any new weight loss plan with your doctor before getting started. A doctor may suggest that losing a pound a week is too much for you.

FAT LOSS VS. MUSCLE LOSS—A COMPLICATION

An unfortunate part of weight loss is that not all the weight you lose comes from fat. You will also lose muscle mass and water weight. As long as you stay hydrated, you don't have to worry about water weight loss, but you want to minimize muscle loss as much as you can.

No matter what, you will lose some muscle as your body adapts to being in a caloric deficit. However, you can prevent muscle loss by not eating too far below your BMR. You also want to avoid high-intensity exercise while dieting unless you're getting adequate protein intake. We'll talk more about nutrition and protein in Chapter 4.

You may get excited when you start seeing the scale move and decide it's a good idea to drop your calorie consumption well below your BMR. You'll probably lose weight if you do this, but you will lose a higher percentage of muscle mass the larger your caloric deficit is. You also risk not getting enough nutrients to stay healthy when you have too large of a caloric deficit. For these reasons, it's best to focus on slow and steady deficits to see long-term results.

WEIGHT LOSS AS A SCIENCE

You can use Excel or any other digital spreadsheet to easily track your average caloric deficit. Using the math in this chapter, you can calculate by which month you will end up at a certain weight level. Fitness tracking apps like Fitbit can calculate your BMR for you too and help keep you on track for your weight loss goal.

Remember that target dates only work when you log your food accurately and use safe numbers for calories burned. Now that you understand how to calculate your BMR and the benefits of logging your food and exercise, let's explore other ways you can use technology to improve your foundational results.

CHAPTER 3

LEVERAGING TECHNOLOGY FOR WEIGHT LOSS

If there's one thing I know, it's that any extra effort in a fitness program will cause people to fall off the wagon.

In this chapter, we're going to talk about the tools and gadgets I've come across to help make losing weight easy, so you stick to the plan. There are a lot of modern conveniences to simplify the process, so let's round out our foundational knowledge here before moving on to the fat freezing protocol.

I've tried various fitness trackers, smartphone apps, and physical devices like Bluetooth scales and measuring tapes. The items I share in this chapter have been tested and work well for improving progress on the *Ice Sculpture Diet*.

For a full list of products I use and recommend throughout this book, check out: icesculpturediet.com/recs.

Let's start by exploring tools that make keeping track of your weight easy.

HOW I FOUGHT WITH BLUETOOTH SCALES UNTIL THEY WON

A few years ago, I started seeing shiny, new Bluetooth scales making their way into the market. At the time, I didn't even have a scale. I weighed myself at the gym whenever I remembered to (bad idea, by the way). You should pick a time each day to weigh yourself consistently. This helps reduce weight fluctuations in your data that naturally happen after eating meals. Consistency also prevents you from just simply forgetting to do it.

When seeing these Bluetooth scales pop up on Amazon, I kept thinking to myself, *Why do these tech companies keep creating unnecessary products? Who would ever need a Bluetooth scale anyway?* I didn't want one and thought buying one was a waste of money. I was wrong.

Everything changed when I decided to get serious with weight loss and needed data to measure my progress. I was getting more active in the fitness world and wanted to track my weight easier, so I decided to give Bluetooth scales a shot. The first time I stepped on one, I was sold.

I learned that Bluetooth scales could sync your weight with apps like Fitbit and Apple Health. Without any extra effort, I had a daily record of my weight over the course of a few months. The best part was that I could see my weight visualized in charts and watch the downward trend happening in my Fitbit app.

Had I been manually entering my weight, I could not have been nearly as accurate as letting the scale log it for me. If you set up your Bluetooth scale correctly (and they're very easy to set up), you will have your weight data synced to your phone whenever you step on it.

Any newer Bluetooth scale should work, but refer back to the link I referenced to see the ones I've tried and tested.

In the data world, we have a saying: "If you want something to change, measure it." For less than thirty dollars, you can monitor your daily and weekly progress easily. You'll have an exportable history of your weight and a lot of other helpful data, including estimated body fat, lean body weight, and water weight. Most of these scale apps also calculate your BMR and Body Mass Index (BMI). BMI is a common factor used in health and fitness studies, so it is useful to know what yours is as a measure of overall health.

When buying a scale, make sure that it can sync with Apple Health, Fitbit, or other smart tracking devices. Like I mentioned earlier, having every-thing in one app makes achieving your goals all that much easier.

Now let's talk about step logging.

HOW FITNESS TRACKERS MOTIVATED ME TO LOSE 35 POUNDS

As I mentioned before, I advocate for a simple approach to exercise. I want people following the *Ice Sculpture Diet* to know they don't have to run 10 miles a week to lose weight.

For now, let's focus on how we can stay motivated to hit our step goals.

To increase the number of calories you burn, I recommended walking 10,000 steps daily. Steps are easily tracked using fitness trackers, making them a great metric for goal-setting.

Fitness trackers are now fairly commonplace and affordable. If you own a Fitbit or an Apple Watch, you're off to a great start. If you aren't sold on getting a fitness tracker, you can check to see if your phone can track steps for you. Many smartphones have step trackers built into them.

I personally like having a separate device for tracking steps. It reminds me that I'm on a mission. Looking at my Fitbit, I'll think, *Holy cow, I haven't hit my steps yet today!* If you are serious about hitting your weight goal, these reminders alone make fitness trackers worth the price.

On a few occasions, I have used my phone to track steps, but I find I often put my phone down and forget to pick it up. Once you start tracking steps, there's nothing worse than walking a few miles only to realize none of them were tracked. You'll know the feeling once you start tracking your steps! The more you track, the more motivated you will be.

FITNESS TRACKERS AND GAMIFICATION

One of the best features of fitness trackers, like an Apple Watch or Fitbit, is that they turn your goal into a game. With the tracker, getting your steps in will be fun!

These apps have motivating notifications and graphics that keep you pushing along toward your ten thousand steps. The more motivation you can get in a weight loss process, the better. Fitbit even sends alerts toward the end of the day if you're close to ten thousand steps but haven't quite hit the goal yet.

FITBIT VS. APPLE WATCH

Now it's time to revisit specific trackers. I've tried a lot of fitness trackers, but I've stuck with Fitbit the longest. Fitbit was one of the first smart step trackers on the market. You can wear most models on your wrist or clip them on your waistband. When you're wearing a Fitbit, it logs your steps via Bluetooth to an app on your smartphone.

Fitbit's app comes with many features, including communities and the ability to add friends. The community aspect is particularly fun when you want to compete with friends or family members for the highest step count in a week. I'm always checking the weekly scores to see if I beat my sisters in our step competitions (sorry Mel and Cristina). That's how serious it gets.

Fitbit also has a food database that allows you to track food intake. At the time of this writing, Apple Health doesn't allow you to log food, but I expect that will change in the future.

If you're not interested in a standalone fitness tracker like Fitbit, the Apple Watch is another multipurpose option for tracking steps. Apple Watches have a lot of great features beyond fitness tracking. You can view your text messages, listen to Audible, and even take a heart ECG. Keep in mind that, with all these features, Apple Watches are more expensive than traditional fitness trackers. If you only plan on using it to track steps, it may not be worth the cost.

If the idea of wearing a fitness tracker doesn't suit you, iPhones track steps by default. You can simply carry your phone on you throughout the day, and you will see your step count in the Apple Health app. This method works as long as you always carry your phone on you.

MONITORING FOOD INTAKE WITH FITNESS TRACKING APPS

Time to revisit food-logging apps. Many soon-to-be dieters I meet are resistant to monitoring their food intake. You might feel unsure about doing this as well. If you trust me on the benefits of food tracking, though, you'll probably be surprised by your own eating habits after one week of tracking.

Remember that food tracking is easy to do now with

apps. You'll need to use some willpower, but staying on top of tracking will make all the difference as you progress toward your goal weight. If you build a habit of tracking your food and understanding your BMR, you will lose weight. It's that simple. So, check out the apps I recommend below and download one now if you haven't already.

MYFITNESSPAL VS. FITBIT FOOD TRACKING

As I mentioned earlier, MyFitnessPal and Fitbit are my top recommendations for food tracking. Their food databases are sourced from nutrition labels and are extensive. Both apps allow you to log almost any type of meal you've eaten, and each has tens of thousands of entries by dedicated weight loss enthusiasts (like yourself).

I was a huge fan of MyFitnessPal until their app increased ad placements. You can pay for a premium membership to get around these ads, but if you already purchased a Fitbit, it probably makes more sense to start with Fitbit's app.

If you have a Fitbit but still prefer MyFitnessPal for food logging, it is possible to connect your MyFitnessPal account with your Fitbit account. This allows you to sync your food logs from MyFitness-Pal over to Fitbit, so you can have both calories eaten and steps visible in a single app.

I synced my logs from MFP for a long time before Fitbit added their own food-logging database. Now I go with the simpler approach, using just Fitbit for tracking all of my fitness data. Along with my Bluetooth scale set to sync, the Fitbit app is now my one-stop shop for weight, step, and food logging.

You can follow my setup or figure out what will work for you. Whatever technology you choose, make it a process you can follow easily. The *Ice Sculpture Diet* is all about removing complications so you can focus on one important thing: hitting your target weight. The more effortless you can make tracking, the easier it will be to reach your goals.

HOW TO MAKE FOOD LOGGING A ROUTINE

If you have never tracked foods before, it can sound challenging. I'm going to flip the script and say that soon—very soon—you might find it is a fun thing to do.

The way I encourage friends and clients to get into food tracking (or any habit) is to try it for a single day. Log what you ate for breakfast. If you log those eggs and toast once, you are off to a great start.

Once you start tracking, you'll begin learning about the foods you eat. You'll see which foods are worth it and which aren't. As you learn a little bit, you'll want to know more. With your growing knowledge of nutrition and calories, you'll be able to make better choices in the future.

LEARNING THROUGH TRACKING

One of the first things I learned when I started tracking food was that avocados have a ton of calories. They are around 230 calories each. Avocados are amazing, but if you eat three of them a day, you're probably going to gain weight. I was eating one a day when I started logging and decided to cut down to half an avocado a day.

By doing this, I could hit my goals and still enjoy the greatest fruit in the world. Without food logging, I would never have known that avocados might be hindering my progress. Food logging teaches you this and more.

So, start with logging food for one day. See what you learn. If you enjoy learning things about life and about yourself, you'll enjoy this process. You may find that something you like to eat can easily fit within your BMR maintenance window. You may find that some other foods are not worth the calories (Kentucky Fried Chicken, anyone?).

After logging food for one day, try expanding that to a week. Once you make it to a week, you'll start to discover things that will amaze you. From that point on, the process of tracking food will take on a life of its own.

HIGH-IMPACT TRACKING

Of all my recommended methods for weight loss, food and exercise logging has the greatest impact on results. It will help you to understand your body and show you how you can achieve your weight loss goal. Losing weight is also about what you learn as you reshape yourself, and you'll learn a lot by logging your food.

You now understand the importance of tracking your calories in and calories out. You learned about Bluetooth scales, fitness trackers, and food-logging apps. Hopefully, you already have some items on your Amazon wish list to help you make progress.

Now, there's one last step to *The Foundation* before moving into *The Freeze*. It's time to make sure you're getting the right amount of nutrients and supplements, at the right times, in order to stay healthy while dieting. Let's move on now to learn what your body needs in order to function optimally while dieting.

CHAPTER 4

NUTRITION

I ate one hundred Chicken McNuggets once. Yes, you read that correctly. I wasn't messing around with that YouTube challenge.

One hundred Chicken McNuggets is about 4,000 calories. Afterward, I felt exactly how you might expect me to feel—terrible. Here's the thing: considering my BMR, I could lose weight if I allowed myself to eat only one hundred Chicken McNuggets every two days. Would that be good for me? No. Would I lose weight? Yes.

This is an extreme example, but it shows that knowing your BMR doesn't give you the full picture of your health. In fact, not understanding nutrition can lead to some devastating results.

In this chapter, we'll talk about macronutrients and how to understand them so you can feel great while following the *Ice Sculpture Diet*. We'll also talk about supplements that will give you a boost for fat loss and overall health. By the end of this chapter, you'll have a basic understanding of nutrition labels and what percentage of your diet should be carbs, fat, and protein.

MACRONUTRIENT OVERVIEW

There are three key macronutrients that make up everything you eat: protein, carbohydrates, and fat. Technically, alcohol counts as a fourth macronutrient. I'm not making that up; alcohol is actually a macronutrient, but it doesn't provide any actual nutrition (although it can be entertaining).

You've probably heard a lot about these three macronutrients before. Here, we'll touch on the basics for each one, so you'll have overall guidelines for what percentage of your food intake should come from each.

PROTEIN

Protein is the building block for muscle. Protein consists of amino acids that your body uses for tissue repair and many other functions. There are 4 calories in every gram of protein. So, if the nutrition label says your protein shake has 30 grams of protein, you can assume it has at least 120 calories.

Protein is very important for maintaining and growing muscle mass. In general, I recommend having around half a gram of protein per pound of body weight. This is especially true if you are strength training and exercising because you need more protein to repair tissue damage. For the *Ice Sculpture Diet*, you should aim to make protein between 20–35 percent of your total calories.

It's important to mention that some diets tell you to go very low carb or very low fat and eat a lot of protein to lose weight. While protein can leave you feeling full, your body will convert excess protein into carbohydrates and, ultimately, store it as fat. The same applies to excess carbohydrates. If you're interested in reading more about that process, Google "protein conversion gluconeogenesis."

CARBOHYDRATES

Carbs, alongside fats, are vilified macronutrients in the dieting community. I'll admit I was against carbohydrates for a long time while I was on the keto diet (high fat, very low carb diet). I used to think that carbohydrates were largely unnecessary as long as you ate enough protein and fat. This was based on some of the popularized ideas surrounding ketogenic diets and the benefits that come from ketones. I've changed my mind since then on this one.

I've found that a moderate amount of carbs is not only good for you but helps keep you sane in a society filled with carb-loaded temptations. Carbs also are needed for balanced hormone production and to replenish glycogen (the fast-acting energy supply) in your muscles. Like protein, carbohydrates also have 4 calories per gram. For the *Ice Sculpture Diet*, I recommend making carbohydrates 35–50 percent of your daily calories. You can aim for the lower end of that percentage, but don't remove them from your diet.

THE REAL CULPRIT: SUGAR

While I recommend a modest amount of carbs, you should keep an eye out for hidden sugar in foods. Sugar is a common carbohydrate and consuming too much of it prevents weight loss. Your carb intake should be coming from low glycemic index rated foods as much as possible. The glycemic index (GI) is a rating scale used to measure the impact of food on your blood sugar levels. Familiarizing yourself with foods that are high on the GI scale will help you learn which foods to avoid.

The issue with high GI foods and sugar is that they spike insulin levels. Insulin signals the body to begin converting calories to fat. On a positive note, insulin is also responsible for signaling the body to replenish carbohydrate stores in the muscles after a hard workout. A little bit of sugar won't kill you, but if you're consuming more than 50 grams a day while dieting, you should cut down your sugar intake. I recommend Stevia or Xylitol as low-calorie alternatives to sugar. Allulose is another natural option that tastes sweet but only has 10 percent of the calories of sugar.

The majority of your carb intake should be from

high-fiber vegetables or breads, low-sugar fruits (like blueberries or strawberries), and the occasional fun snack. If you're still drinking non-diet sodas or sweet teas, scan one of them into your food-logging app. You'll see how much sugar these drinks have, which will probably convince you to stop drinking them (or at least to stop drinking them so often).

Calories from soda or sweet drinks are a dieter's worst enemy because they don't make you feel full. They also spike your insulin within thirty minutes of drinking them. The carbohydrates you eat should help you feel satisfied, so aim for those high-fiber ones mentioned above. This will make it easier to feel full longer throughout the day.

FAT

Fat is the last key macronutrient, and it is much more important than you think. For a long time, high-fat foods were blamed for the obesity epidemic in the United States. Today, those beliefs are being questioned with the success of high-fat, low-carb diets. Many people are seeing great results on high-fat diets, so what gives?

Well, studies are showing that carbs and sugar may be more of a culprit for weight gain than fat. Like I mentioned previously, consuming sugar or high glycemic index foods causes your body to release insulin. In turn, your body goes into fat storage mode and converts carbohydrates into fat.

Fat, as a macronutrient, doesn't deserve as much of the negative reputation it has. Your body uses dietary fat to produce vital hormones. Fat is also needed for your brain and heart to function properly. To ensure these vital organs are working effectively, keep some fat in your diet.

HOW FAT MUCH SHOULD YOU CONSUME?

Out of the three primary macronutrients, fat is the only one that doesn't have 4 calories per gram; it has 9 calories per gram. Many people look at fat's higher calorie count per gram as a bad thing, but because fat has more calories per gram, it is also more satiating. So, if you eat foods that have some fat in them, you will feel full longer.

Feeling full for as long as you can throughout the day will help you eat less. So, I recommend setting fat intake between 15–25 percent of your daily calories. Be careful, though, because a small amount of fat can have more calories than you might think (remember the avocados?).

MACRONUTRIENT CONSUMPTION GUIDELINES

The above guidelines are not strict rules. They are general suggestions to follow so that your nutrition doesn't go out of whack while dieting. A simple rule to remember is that carbs should make up the highest percentage of your total calories but no more than 50 percent of your total calories. Protein consumption should be second-highest, especially if you are strength training. Fat should be the lowest, but you still want to keep healthy fats, like avocado oil and salmon (also a good source of protein), in your diet.

Many books dive deeper into macronutrient balance. I recommend reading *The Primal Blueprint* by Mark Sisson, a paleo-focused nutrition book, if you want to go deeper into this subject. Like with other health changes, you should speak with your doctor before making major changes to your diet.

VEGETABLES AND THE BEAUTY OF FIBER

Now that you are more familiar with the major macronutrients, let's talk a little bit about vegetables. Vegetables are loaded with nutrients, and I highly recommend making them a part of your daily food intake. To take it a step further, try focusing on vegetables that are high in fiber. Some of these include broccoli, cauliflower, asparagus, and celery.

By eating a lot of high-fiber vegetables, you will feel full while consuming very few calories. Fiber fills up your stomach and helps clear out your intestines. You want to avoid or limit starchy vegetables like potatoes, which are higher in calories and often higher on the GI scale. These high-carb vegetables will ultimately spike your insulin levels, so eat them in moderation.

THE TWO TYPES OF FIBER

You will typically find two types of fiber on nutrition labels: soluble fiber and insoluble fiber.

Soluble fiber is fiber that dissolves in water. Insoluble fiber does not dissolve in water. The good news is that insoluble fiber, even though it's counted as calories on a nutrition label, does not actually get digested by the body. It simply passes through. In other words, insoluble fiber will add very few calories, if any, to your body. Fiber also helps you feel full, so eat as much insoluble fiber as you can.

NET CARBS—A GREAT SIGN

When you look at the packaging for newer protein bars or other health-conscious snacks, you may see "net carbs" written out. Net carbs are the total carbohydrates in the item, minus the carbohydrates from fiber (both types). Companies usually call out their net carb amounts so that consumers can easily see that the item is low in carbs when you exclude fiber. This net carbs label can make it easy for you to find snacks that won't spike your insulin.

Brands that label net carbs on their products also tend to include more protein in their recipes. Their target market is usually health-conscious eaters, so seeing net carbs written out is a shortcut for identifying more diet-friendly snacks. Look for protein bars, cereals (I love Magic Spoon brand), or other treats that have net carb counts below 13 grams or so. These will help keep you satisfied while snacking, without breaking your calorie bank or spiking insulin.

FIBER SUMMARY

With all that said above, the takeaway should be to eat as much insoluble fiber as you can.

Broccoli and cauliflower are perfect here because they're packed with vitamins, nutrients, and insoluble fiber. Many people also enjoy eating celery as a snack. These three vegetables, when eaten with lunch or dinner, will leave you feeling full and satisfied.

WHAT ABOUT FRUITS?

Fruits have a lot of vitamins, but unfortunately, modern fruits are cultivated to have more natural sugar too. I know what you're thinking. *But it's good sugar!* Sorry to be the bearer of bad news, but fructose (the sugar found in fruits) is no different than table sugar. Some studies have even shown that fructose spikes insulin levels more than table sugar does.

I don't want you to go throwing out all your fruit,

though. Eating some fruit here and there won't hurt you, and it provides a valuable sweet treat when dieting. That said, let's take a look at fruit juice drinks like orange juice to understand how concentrated fruit sugars affect our bodies.

ORANGE JUICE NUTRITION = OUCH

If you look up the nutrition facts for a glass of orange juice, you'll see that it has roughly 22 grams of sugar. For reference, a packet of sugar used in coffee holds between 3 to 5 grams of sugar. So, drinking a glass of orange juice is equivalent to drinking four to five packets of sugar.

Yes, OJ is loaded with Vitamin C, but no more than what you can get from a vitamin C supplement that has 0 calories. If you drink a glass of orange juice with your breakfast like the TV ads suggest, your insulin will spike. These spikes will begin the fat storage process and negatively affect your weight loss efforts. The lesson: avoid OJ if you can.

CHEATING WITH FRUIT

Do I sometimes cheat and eat fruit or drink fruit

juices? Yes, even with mimosas during brunch every few months. It's all about balance. Understanding nutrition is not meant to make you feel guilty for what you eat. It should give you awareness of the calorie and sugar content that is often overlooked in common foods. Once you're aware, it's up to you to decide if there are better alternatives for the calories in your BMR bank account. You can spend it however you want.

Now that we've touched on fruits and vegetables, let's talk about some other ways to get nutrients through vitamin and supplement additions.

VITAMINS AND OTHER SUPPLEMENTS

When changing your diet, it's easy to miss out on key vitamins you might otherwise get from eating random foods. In this section, I'll share a few supplements I take daily to stay healthy.

MULTIVITAMIN SUPPLEMENT

This one is obvious, but everyone should be taking some form of a multivitamin. The one-a-day vitamins are fine, but there are much higher quality vitamins available in powder capsule form if you want to get better absorption.

Generally, the compressed tablet multivitamins are not as bioavailable as powder capsules. Bioavailability is just a way of saying how much of the vitamin is actually absorbed in the bloodstream. Higher-end vitamins often go through different processing to make the nutrients more easily absorbed during digestion. If you want a higher-end vitamin, I recommend Thorne RX powder capsule vitamins. If you're just looking to get started with something, try something simple like Amazon Elements multivitamins.

There are some key differences between men's and women's branded vitamins. The main difference is in iron content. Men don't need a lot of excess iron, which is why it's kept out. At certain levels, iron is actually detrimental to your health.

One interesting fact I learned over the years is that donating blood is a great way for men to reduce iron levels. If you're interested in learning more about this, there's an entire book on the subject called *Dumping Iron* by P.D. Mangan.

Women's multivitamins include more iron because women ovulate, which reduces their iron levels. Prenatal vitamins are also specifically designed for pregnant women and include more DHA fats (more on DHA later).

Besides iron, ensure that your multivitamin has some support for vitamin D levels. Many people are vitamin D deficient without knowing it due to lack of sun exposure. You can also buy a separate vitamin D supplement if you're concerned about getting a higher dose. Vitamin D supplements are usually inexpensive.

FISH OIL SUPPLEMENT

There are many studies showing the benefits of fish oil. It is great for your health, and some studies have shown it reduces the risk of fatal diseases, heart attacks, stroke, and even dementia.

That said, some fish oil mixes are better than others. I highly recommend looking at the EPA and DHA Omega-3 fat levels in your fish oil supplement before purchasing. EPA and DHA should be listed out on the label. DHA is very important for brain health and development; the more of it, the better. EPA helps offset cellular inflammation that can occur from consuming too many Omega-6 fatty acids. The daily fish oil serving I take is three soft gels, which contain around 1200 mg of EPA and 900 mg of DHA. If EPA and DHA are not listed, look for another brand or ask their product support for detailed information.

Some fish oil supplements boast high Omega fat content, but it comes from Omega-6 fats. Omega-6 fats, in high quantities, can lead to inflammation in the body. Inflammation is the body's response to an irritant of some form and causes problems for your health. Aim to get as much Omega-3 fats as you can while minimizing Omega-6 fats. Most fish oil or krill oil supplements will mention the Omega fat content levels on their label. If they don't, go for a different brand with more Omega-3s.

For a specific list of fish oil supplements and other vitamins I take, check out the full list of my recommendations here: icesculpturediet.com/recs.

CURCUMIN EXTRACT

Most people I meet have never taken curcumin or turmeric extract. Many studies have concluded that both provide a host of benefits for your heart, circulation, and even digestion.

I take around 1 gram of curcumin extract per day. Afterward, I rest knowing it is helping my body and more than likely extending my life. It's relatively inexpensive for the health benefits it provides. Do your body a favor and add this to your daily stack. It's one of my secrets for good health.

GREEN TEA EXTRACT (ENERGY + WEIGHT LOSS!)

I've been taking green tea extract for its health benefits for years. Numerous studies show that taking green tea extract has been correlated to weight loss in double-blind (read: properly performed) studies. Green tea is filled with polyphenols, which are healthy antioxidants. An extracted version is just a little bit more concentrated and potent.

You could also aim to drink a glass or two of green tea each day if you don't want to purchase the extract capsules. The extracted form can make your life easier, as it is the equivalent of up to 5 to 10 cups of tea in terms of nutrients and health benefits. Take it in the morning since it does have some caffeine that could keep you up if you take it later in the afternoon.

THE IMPORTANCE OF FEELING FULL

One of your primary goals when eating on a diet should be satiation (feeling full). I mentioned earlier that proteins and fats tend to keep you full longer. Fiber helps in this area too. Simple carbs (sugar), on the other hand, could have you feeling hungry within an hour.

Feeling full makes it easier to stay within your BMR calorie threshold because, obviously, you'll be much less likely to snack. It is possible to hack how full we feel using meal timing as well. Let's talk about that now.

INTERMITTENT FASTING FOR A SATIATION BOOST

The concept of intermittent fasting has become very popular recently. I use it, and I recommend incorporating it into your protocol, so you can reap the benefits of shorter eating windows.

When you practice intermittent fasting (IF), the idea is to eat your meals within a specific time window and fast (don't eat) outside of that window. This is fairly easy to stick with, given that half of the fast happens while you're asleep.

The main benefit of IF is that you can skip a meal (usually breakfast) without feeling hungry. This means you're consuming fewer calories without really noticing it. You can do this while still getting enough nutrients to be healthy too. Fasting has also been shown to increase autophagy, which is the cleanup of old or damaged cells throughout the body. Autophagy is a natural process that keeps the body functioning well, so increasing autophagy is a good thing.

A typical IF schedule involves an eight-hour eating window and a sixteen-hour fasting window. Since it is easier to fast overnight while you're sleeping, many people eat from noon to 8:00 p.m. and skip breakfast altogether.

You can start IF by eating a light snack early in the day, but the farther you can push out your window for eating, the more effective IF is. I eat a light breakfast, usually more of a snack, around 11:00 a.m. on most days. My feeding window is generally from 11:00 a.m. to 7:00 p.m.

TIMING FOR INTERMITTENT FASTING

You can be flexible with the sixteen-hour time range. Doing a fourteen- or fifteen-hour fast has similar benefits for weight loss, as long as you don't make it any shorter. The goal is to shrink your eating window while feeling full for most of the time you are awake.

If you normally eat breakfast at 6:00 a.m., you are probably hungry again by noon. Having a habit of eating when you wake up actually puts your mind in a routine of eating, even if you aren't hungry. Alternatively, if you start fasting at 8:00 p.m., you will feel a little bit hungry by 10:00 a.m. but not starving by noon.

This meal timing helps you feel full for a longer period of time, naturally causing you to eat less.

If you're looking to read more about intermittent fasting protocols, my favorite book on the subject is *The Leangains Method* by Martin Berkhan.

MEAL TIMING SUMMARY

In summary, you can improve your results on the *Ice Sculpture Diet* by using intermittent fasting to time your meals.

Start with a light breakfast around 10:00 or 11:00 a.m. (200–500 calories), have a medium-sized lunch between noon and 2:00 p.m., and then eat a heavier dinner around 6:00 p.m. Before 8:00 p.m. hits, you might have a protein shake to maintain muscle mass and hold you over until the next day. After 8:00 p.m., call it quits.

If you try out intermittent fasting for a day and then for a week, you might find that IF starts to feel very natural and effortless.

KEEPING YOUR MUSCLE MASS WHILE DIETING

Eating at your BMR level while walking 10,000 steps a day should produce enough of a caloric deficit for you to lose a good amount of fat each week without burning off a lot of muscle.

Shrinking muscle mass, while expected during a diet, is generally not a good thing for overall strength. Fortunately, there are a couple of ways to minimize muscle loss:

1. Eat at your BMR level, or no less than 70 percent of total calories burned, if you are exercising
2. If you do notice muscle loss, you can take advantage of fat freezing, outlined in Chapter 6, to increase fat loss while adding back some more calories to your intake

You can always gain muscle back once you hit your fat reduction goal. Don't let muscle loss distract you too much from your target. Keep focused on weight loss, and you can learn about muscle gain later using the bonus chapter at the end of this book.

WRAPPING UP NUTRITION

You now have a foundational understanding of how your body works and the science behind weight loss.

Since you've read through this far, take a moment to congratulate yourself.

There's a lot more to come, but let's review what you've learned in this chapter.

You saw, from the McNuggets example at the beginning, that it is theoretically possible to lose weight while eating whatever you want. That isn't always healthy, though.

To keep your health in check, aim for the macronutrient ratios described in this chapter (20–35 percent protein, 40–50 percent carbohydrates, and 15–25 percent fat). Include insoluble fiber in your diet so that you feel satiated. Add vitamins and supplements like fish oil and curcumin to your diet to improve your overall health. Time your meals, using intermittent fasting, so that you can easily feel full during the day with calories to spare. Finally, try to maintain as much muscle mass as possible by eating no less than 70 percent of your calorie expenditure for the day.

You've made it through *The Foundation*. Everything going forward builds off the nutrition plan laid out here, and there's a lot more to come. Now it's time to go to the next level for fat reduction and the one you're probably most excited to learn about: fat freezing. If you're ready to break through plateaus and reshape your body, turn to *The Freeze* to learn the technique that changed my dieting routine forever.

PART II

THE FREEZE

CHAPTER 5

THE SCIENCE BEHIND FAT FREEZING

"We are so successful at being comfortable that comfort has become the enemy of our success."

—WIM HOF

What you learned in the previous chapters is enough to help you lose weight on its own. It's the basis for all weight loss. For many years, I followed what was written in *The Foundation* and saw great, short-term success. Then, I discovered a new way to remove a crazy amount of fat from targeted areas of my body.

Once I built a routine around this method, with *The Foundation* to start, the results I achieved were fantastic. I gained a new way of looking at fat loss, and you will too. In this chapter, I'll share with you the background behind that technique before jumping into the *Ice Sculpture Freeze Routine*.

Let's dive into the latest in fat reduction methods: at-home fat freezing.

Many people haven't heard about fat freezing as a method for targeting and reducing fat. Others have heard about it but didn't know it was possible to do easily at home. The first reaction I get when I explain this technique from the *Ice Sculpture Diet* is usually doubt. *You can freeze fat and make it disappear?* You might be thinking this too.

I was also skeptical about fat freezing until I added it to my overall plan and started seeing my abs again. The results were so good that I kept it in my weekly routine for maintenance, even after I had a six-pack. After experiencing this success, I knew I had to share my experience with others. In case it isn't clear yet, fat freezing works. Let's talk about how.

HOW FAT FREEZING WORKS

There's a method to the madness. You don't want to simply place ice packs on random parts of your body. In fact, you will hurt yourself if you do this. What I'm going to show you in this chapter is a safe way to use ice wraps to reduce fat. I call this process fat freezing, but the technical term is cold-induced fat apoptosis (CIFA).

I remember first hearing about CIFA back in 2017 and thinking to myself, *There is no possible way this could work, or I would've heard about it by now.* I'm grateful I was willing to open my mind and research more. What I discovered ended up being the one thing that worked for getting rid of that stubborn belly fat that I had since I was a kid.

CIFA works for one simple reason: fat cells freeze at a higher temperature than surrounding skin and other tissue. If you can create an environment where fat cells freeze without affecting the skin, muscle, or other cells near the fat, you can target the fat closest to the skin for an overall reduction in fat.

It's important to know that there are two types of

fat in the body. There's visceral fat, which is the fat stored deeper in your body, surrounding your organs. Then, there's subcutaneous fat, or the fat that is closest to the surface of your skin.

If you follow the steps outlined in *The Foundation*, you will be reducing both visceral and subcutaneous fat. In *The Freeze*, we're looking to specifically reduce subcutaneous fat using fat freezing methods. Fat freezing is the icing on the cake for this plan; it allows us to get leaner even when the scale isn't moving.

I'm going to walk you through the entire *Ice Sculpture Freeze Routine* soon. You'll be able to easily follow along and see results using this and *The Foundation*. First, let's look at how CIFA was discovered and the science behind it so that we understand our options.

HOW CIFA WAS DISCOVERED

In 1970, two doctors, Dr. Mark Oren and Dr. Ervin Epstein, discovered and coined the term "popsicle panniculitis."

Oren and Epstein were investigating the case of a

toddler who was brought into their office. The child had developed dimples shortly after eating a popsicle. They hypothesized that the popsicle was held against the infant's inner cheek long enough that it damaged the fat cells in the infant's cheek. This left the child with a cold-induced dimple, hence the name "popsicle" panniculitis. Panniculitis, by the way, is the medical term for when bumps form in subcutaneous fat.

Oren and Epstein coined the term but didn't do much else with their discovery. Years passed before other researchers began wondering if the method could be used for more targeted fat loss. Today, we know of several methods for freezing fat off the body.

What's amazing about fat freezing is that it causes fat cells to be permanently removed from your body. Fat cells rarely die on their own. Once they are created, they either shrink or grow based on your diet. Fat freezing gives your body a way to remove these cells entirely. Once fat cells are frozen long enough, your body naturally begins to remove them through its cleanup process.

Your body may make more fat cells if your diet isn't

in check, though. This is why the book starts with *The Foundation* to keep you prepared.

HOW TO FREEZE FAT—THE TRUE METHODS

You can freeze fat using professional services or using online products at home. Professional services are available in the price range of $500 to $2,000 per visit. These visits are highly effective and work in as little as one to two sessions. If that price tag shocks you, know that you can also freeze fat at home, often for less than $100. The at-home process is what we'll be using in the *Ice Sculpture Freeze Routine*. While the process at home is not as quick or as well-studied, my personal experience and the testimonials of others online show that it works very well. I'll talk about both options in this chapter before moving on.

If you are looking to go the professional route, I'll share my personal experience with CoolSculpting® first. If this method is outside of your budget, feel free to skip to the at-home fat freezing section that follows. What you read below is only my opinion and understanding of the CoolSculpting® procedure as I went through it.

If you want to learn more about the most well-known professional fat freezing service, please visit Coolsculpting.com. I am in no way affiliated with CoolSculpting® or its services. What you read here is simply my personal experience after trying out the procedure.

COOLSCULPTING® FAT FREEZING PROCEDURE

A fat freezing book wouldn't be complete without mention of CoolSculpting®. This is a professional service that varies in price depending on where you get it done. I tried CoolSculpting® on two separate occasions before I got serious about dieting, and the results were impressive.

I lost a significant amount of visible fat from key areas (my abdomen and flank area). I found that one visit was enough to see results, but if you have a lot of fat to lose, you will likely need multiple sessions.

After having one session and seeing the results, it's very tempting to return for a second visit. I say this because I ended up going for a second session after seeing the first round of results.

HOW DOES COOLSCULPTING® WORK?

Most clinics offer a free consultation to discuss the procedure with you and outline target areas before booking the freezing session. During treatment, the CoolSculpting® application device is placed on the desired target area for around thirty minutes per treatment. It creates a vacuum seal to pull fat closer and uses cooling technology to freeze fat. The device itself is temperature regulated. It keeps a precise temperature to ensure that your fat is being frozen while your skin tissue is protected.

Before securing the device on the target area, the technician will put a specialized gel cover on the treatment area to protect it. Following each thirty-minute treatment, the technician will massage the area for around five to eight minutes. Massaging increases the removal of frozen fat cells from your body, so it's important.

The technician usually leaves the room while the applicator is on since you're sitting still for about thirty minutes. If the applicator begins to slip for any reason, the technician receives an alert from the machine to come back. This happened to me during one of my sessions but was not really a cause for concern. My technician returned and adjusted the applicator a bit, and we were good to go.

MY COOLSCULPTING® EXPERIENCE

The two sessions I had were around three hours long each. During these appointments, I had several treatment areas done. The technician was knowledgeable and friendly during my pre-treatment consultation. She pinpointed areas to target, set expectations, and provided guidance for what to do after the procedure.

During my CoolSculpting® sessions, the target areas felt extremely cold, as expected. This feeling lasted for about five minutes, and then the area started to feel numb. After this, you don't really feel the area at all, and it is very manageable. I brought headphones with me and listened to an audiobook while the machine did its job. All in all, it was a simple experience with great results.

I did not lose any weight after CoolSculpting®, but I certainly lost visible fat. I'll admit that I did CoolSculpting® at a time when I was not focusing deeply on my health. So, while I definitely lost fat,

I was missing out on the foundation for weight loss. Once I followed the diet details outlined in Part I of this book and combined it with fat freezing at home, I achieved 9 percent body fat for the first time in my life. This is why it's important to follow the entire outline of the *Ice Sculpture Diet*.

HOW LONG DOES IT TAKE TO SEE RESULTS?

The results from CoolSculpting® are not instant. It can take two to three months before all the frozen fat cells are cleared from your body, but you may begin to see results within four weeks following your session.

As with any fat freezing technique, it takes time for your body to flush out the affected fat cells. I started seeing visible results within thirty to sixty days.

PROS OF COOLSCULPTING®

- Single-day, high-impact sessions
- FDA approved for specific areas (very well researched)
- Professional service with trained technicians
- Documented patient success (it works)

CONS OF COOLSCULPTING®

The only real con of CoolSculpting® is the price, which makes it unaffordable for some people. Some users have also reported extended numbness in the treatment areas.

If you can afford it, I highly recommend following Part I and III of this book while using CoolSculpting® when you hit a plateau in your weight loss.

That said, you don't have to go this route. Let's talk about the options I regularly use now to freeze fat at home.

AT-HOME FAT FREEZING WITH ICE WRAPS

It is possible to freeze fat from the comfort of your home. I do it regularly now and will recommend it in our freezing routine to follow. There are a lot of sketchy fat freezing products out there. I've researched and used several products that stand above the rest in the market. I'll outline which ones I use in the next chapter. For now, let's talk about the pros and cons of at-home fat freezing.

HOW DO THESE ICE WRAPS WORK?

At-home freezing products usually work by placing ice packs into a specially made belt or wrap. The wrap is designed to protect your skin from direct contact with the ice packs. They're often designed to be worn for between thirty minutes to one hour at a time. These ice wraps are designed to be comfortable and allow you to do other activities while they're on, though I recommend sitting while using them. Sitting during use ensures you won't heat up the target areas too quickly, causing the ice to melt.

If frozen properly, specialty ice wraps should bring your fat down to a temperature that causes some fat cells to freeze and die off. That said, some research questions the effectiveness of these belts, noting the belts' inability to guarantee a low enough temperature for the required time needed to freeze fat.

I have personally experienced success with these belts, and many reviews match my experience. I recommend ice wraps for the *Ice Sculpture Diet* because I've seen them work. Some fat freezing products also offer a guaranteed test period, so you can judge their effectiveness for yourself and return them if you're unsatisfied.

PROS OF FREEZING FAT WITH ICE WRAPS

- Use from home while doing normal activities
- Much cheaper than professional or surgical fat reduction options
- You can target several areas on your body with a single wrap
- Wraps can be used repeatedly for multiple sessions
- Generally great customer support for these products

CONS OF ICE WRAPS AND BELTS

- It takes many more sessions to have an impact (two to three times a week for several weeks)
- Their temperature will fluctuate due to the ice packs melting
- Ice packs can take up a lot of space in the freezer (I have a whole shelf of ice packs now)
- Ice packs can leak if you tighten too much (some companies will replace these packs)

HOW LONG DOES IT TAKE TO SEE RESULTS?

You will see visible results from fat freezing within four weeks to three months. Though the fat may be frozen immediately, your body takes up to three months to remove the affected fat cells from the target area.

I like to say the impact is immediate because some fat cells stop functioning after your very first session. Any freezing session will have a lasting impact. If you use ice wraps two to three times a week, each session will add to your overall results as long as the ice packs are fully frozen.

HOW CAN I MAXIMIZE MY FAT REDUCTION?

Performing a single ice wrap session won't make a large difference on your physique. The process I'm going to outline in the next chapter takes about two to three applications a week, for about thirty minutes to one hour at a time.

Follow this protocol, along with monitoring your calories, to ensure both subcutaneous and visceral fat are being affected. If you stick with fat freezing for even four weeks, I think you'll be very happy with the results. If you stick with it for six months, you will be amazed by the end.

A DISCLAIMER: FAT FREEZING IS NOT RIGHT FOR EVERYONE

Fat freezing is safe for most people. Of course, you want to follow the product instructions and never let ice packs directly touch unprotected skin. This could lead to frostbite. Quality fat freezing products prevent direct contact with specialty material. The products I recommend later are designed to protect you while still effectively cooling fat.

This said, I am not a doctor. Anyone with existing health conditions should consult a medical professional before attempting any diet or fat freezing process outlined here.

From my research, people with the following disorders should not attempt fat freezing:

- Cryoglobulinemia
- Paroxysmal cold hemoglobinuria
- Cold agglutinin disease

If you have any pre-existing medical conditions or concerns not covered here, please reach out to your doctor before proceeding.

ONWARD TO FAT FREEZING

Now you understand how fat freezing was discovered and the process behind it. You also learned about both professional fat freezing services and at-home options that are available.

Next up, I will outline the exact process I used to lose inches from my waist, legs, and back—all from the comfort of my sofa. I even used fat freezing while writing this book. (I'm using an ice wrap now as I write this sentence.) It's your turn to learn and follow the *Ice Sculpture Diet Freeze Routine*. Turn now to learn how to experience enhanced fat loss for yourself.

CHAPTER 6

USING ICE WRAPS TO CHISEL YOUR BODY

As I'm writing the introduction to this chapter, fat is permanently being removed from my body. How is this happening? Ice wraps.

I'm wearing one right now around my abs. I've been using this routine two to three times a week for the past three months, and I've lost several inches off of my waist. Of course, I'm following everything else you've read in the previous chapters, but the *Ice Sculpture Freeze Routine* you're about to learn is a motivation like no other.

Sure, you might get a few odd looks from your friends when you tell them you're using ice wraps to reduce fat. When something sounds crazy, I investigate it, so I can decide for myself. I encourage you to do the same while reading this chapter and preparing for your first freeze. You will be glad you did when you show up looking great at the beach next summer.

There are a lot of products out there for fat freezing, many of which do not work. The ones I recommend here do work and often have a money-back guarantee. You can try the freeze wraps to experience the results for yourself. If you follow what I outline, you won't be returning anything because you should see your waist shrinking after a few weeks.

STUBBORN FAT AND HOW TO GET RID OF IT WITH ICE

Like it or not, you can't tell your body to burn fat from specific areas when exercising or dieting. On some days, your body will decide that burning fat off of your abs is a good idea, while on other days, it will burn thigh fat or visceral fat.

Until fat freezing was discovered, the only real

option to lose targeted fat was to keep dieting and hope for the best or to get liposuction. Now, with fat freezing, we have the ability to target where we want to lose fat from our bodies.

Simply use the products I'll mention here and follow the routine provided on your target area. You should begin seeing a reduction in fat within four weeks, while the full effect can take up to three months.

THE BASICS OF AT-HOME FAT FREEZING

At-home fat freezing is really quite simple, but you need to be dedicated to the routine to see results. In a nutshell, we'll be following a two to three session per week freezing protocol. You'll decide on the target areas, but you'll always be able to move to new target areas after you see reductions in one.

The target areas I focused on were my stomach, thighs, and back. Yours may be different. If you target locations with a larger amount of fat, you should see a larger reduction in fat. This is because locations with more fat have a larger surface area available for the freezing product to impact.

If you are already lean, the freezing protocol can still help you. I've used it on my arms, which were fairly lean, to increase vascularity in my biceps. I continued to use ice wraps even after I hit 9 percent body fat. By doing so, I saw the veins appear again in my arms and lower abs, giving me a great vascular definition.

PRODUCTS I RECOMMEND FOR AT-HOME FAT REDUCTION

To begin, you'll need to get some ice packs. It is possible to get results using just ice packs and cloth, but I do not recommend this approach. Using a do-it-yourself approach with ice and cloth makes it very difficult to keep things safe. If you do go this route, you can't let the ice packs directly touch your skin, but again I don't recommend it.

MY FAVORITE FAT-FREEZING WRAPS

I recommend purchasing a product specifically designed for targeted fat reduction using ice. There are a few great products on the market, but I've had awesome success using the Isavera brand abdominal wrap and Isavera thigh wraps.

The Isavera wraps come with specialty gel ice packs that maintain their temperature longer than regular ice packs. These ice wraps also have cooling slots for each ice pack that help protect your skin while freezing fat. The wraps are adjustable with Velcro, so they will easily fit specific areas of your body. I find these wraps very comfortable to wear for an hour at a time.

CHECK THE REVIEWS AND TESTIMONIALS

At the time of this writing, you can take one look at the reviews for Isavera and see the success that customers are having with the product. That's what initially piqued my interest in the wraps, and I was extremely satisfied with my own results. The wraps also came with a money-back guarantee, which I ultimately didn't use because I found them so effective.

If you do go and purchase them but aren't seeing results, reach out to customer support to get help. Their customer service is top-notch. You can't really go wrong with these.

From this point forward, I'm going to outline a

freezing protocol using the Isavera wraps. You can substitute the Isavera wraps for another fat-freezing product if you chose a different one. Just be aware that there are a lot of fake fat-freezing products on Amazon that produce poor results, so choose wisely. In picking out a product, look for satisfaction guarantees and check to see that customers are actually experiencing results using the product.

Before moving on to the freezing protocol, make sure you have something ready to use for your freezing sessions. Most of the products I've mentioned so far (and other favorites and potential discounts) can be found here: icesculpturediet. com/recs.

Now that we have our freezing tools figured out, let's talk about how to use them most effectively.

THE *ICE SCULPTURE DIET* FREEZE PROTOCOL

As part of our fat-loss plan, we're going to freeze for two to three sessions a week. Some people like to focus on multiple target areas to start. I recommend focusing on a single target area first so that you can build up a routine. If you're already prepared to stick to the routine, feel free to rotate between different target areas.

Each session should be about one hour long, so pick a time where you'll be able to sit for at least an hour. Again, I suggest sitting while wearing the ice wraps because other activities may cause your body to heat up and melt the ice packs faster. I also recommend turning these sessions into a habitual practice so that your mind gets used to this and it becomes easy. Pick a specific hour of the day that you can perform this routine for two to three days a week.

The ice packs need to be fully frozen before use. This means that when you first get your ice packs, you should freeze them for at least twenty-four hours. The first time I attempted fat freezing, I waited just five hours for the ice packs to freeze. This wasn't enough time, and the ice packs melted halfway through the session. If you use partially frozen ice packs, you're not going to get the results you're expecting. I recommend setting your freezer temperature slightly colder than usual, especially when you first start using the ice wraps. This way, you're guaranteed the highest impact during each freezing session.

Take the ice packs out of the freezer and place them into the safety slots that are available on your ice wrap. Make sure you aren't holding the ice packs for very long, as the heat from your hand will begin to melt them. Try holding the ice packs from the edges when inserting them into the wrap.

When putting the wraps on, tighten the wrap as close to the skin as you can. I find that sometimes these products leave a bit of a gap due to the way the pockets are sewn into the wraps. Try to tighten the belt enough that you minimize this gap.

One trick is to find an extra belt from your closet and wrap it around the outside of the ice wrap. This can help to ensure full contact of the wrap on your body. Just make sure the outer belt isn't too tight, as too much pressure can cause the ice packs to break.

The first time you attempt this freezing protocol, try doing it for thirty minutes. Use your first freezing session to experience what the cold feels like before using any of the enhancement tips I recommend here. If thirty minutes seems easy, then continue for the full hour. The cool feeling will only last for about seven to ten minutes before your skin and body adapt. So, if you're feeling cold for the first seven minutes, try to hang in there for a little bit longer. Your body will adapt, and the results will be worth it.

After your first thirty minutes or one hour are up, take off the wraps and set them aside. You'll want to dry off any condensation on the ice packs before putting them back in the freezer. If there is enough space in your freezer, you can put the entire wrap in (keeping the ice packs in the wrap). That said, you may find putting just the ice packs in the freezer, without the belt, helps them freeze faster and more completely.

After your freezing session, there's one more step to improve fat reduction and circulation.

MASSAGING AFTER FAT FREEZING

Once you've worn your wrap for an hour, you'll have partially frozen fat cells underneath your skin. If the fat cells reach a cool-enough temperature, your body will begin removing them over the next few weeks.

Some of these fat cells will naturally die after freezing, but others may warm up again and "come back to life." Massaging the area helps increase blood circulation and potentially breaks up additional fat cells.

EXTRA TOOLS FOR MASSAGING

Isavera wraps come with a small massaging tool to help increase circulation in the focus area. You can also manually massage the area using lotion for five minutes. Applying lotion to the area first makes it much easier for you to massage the cool surface.

If you want to get the maximum effect, I recommend using a percussion massager. A lot of people use these for muscle recovery after a hard workout. They also effectively increase circulation following a fat freezing session. If you use this kind of massager on your abs, be sure to flex your core. Otherwise, the massage will be painful.

Percussion massagers can be a little pricey, ranging between $150 to $500. I received the one I recommend as a gift (thanks, team!), and it is priced at around $200. If you plan to also use it for massaging muscles after you work out, it's worth the price because it feels amazing.

After you massage all frozen areas for around five minutes, your freezing session is complete.

WRAPPING UP

You've learned a lot in the last two chapters about how to use ice to reduce fat. In Chapter 5, you learned the science of fat freezing and how it was discovered. In this chapter, I shared with you the steps I used to reshape my body and break free from plateaus.

Let's do a quick recap of the important points from this chapter.

- Fat freezing works best with specially designed products
- Never place an ice pack directly on your skin
- Look for a product that has specific slots for ice packs to protect your skin
- Look for products that have excellent testimonials since there are a lot of ineffective products out there

- Wear your ice wraps for thirty minutes to one hour per session
- Aim for two to three freezing sessions a week
- Massage the target area, following an ice wrap session, to increase circulation and enhance your fat reduction in that area
- Remember that it takes four to eight weeks (or longer) for fat cells to be cleared from your body, so be patient

If you have yet to purchase ice wraps online, see a full list of the ones I use (and potential discounts) here: icesculpturediet.com/recs.

Now you are equipped with everything you need for targeted fat reduction using fat freezing. You're ready to become a chiseled ice sculpture. Before we move on to Part III, I'm going to share a case study from my own experience on the full *Ice Sculpture Diet* plan, so you can see how all of this works when put together.

CHAPTER 7

ICE SCULPTURE DIET CASE STUDY

You've received a lot of information up to this point, and you might be wondering what this entire plan looks like when it's done right for a few months. So, here's a complete case study of how I lost 35 pounds using all the advice you've read so far. I'll also share some tips I wish I knew before I started the plan.

Keep in mind, roughly four months of this case study took place during the full COVID-19 lockdown, when gyms were closed and outdoor activities were limited. Getting steps was not easy. Thankfully, I didn't have to go to the gym to see this weight come off.

THE STARTING STATS

Start Date: Jan. 1, 2020

Starting Weight: 192.6 pounds

Starting BMR: 1,800 calories

THE ENDING STATS

End Date: May 31, 2020

Ending Weight: 157.6 pounds

Ending BMR: 1,720 calories (BMR decreases as you lose weight)

Total Weight Loss: 35 pounds

BEFORE PICTURE

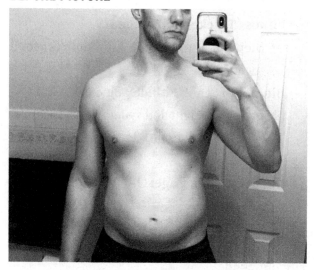

AFTER PICTURE

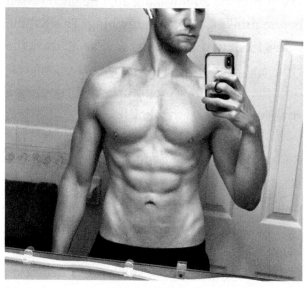

THE TECHNOLOGY

- **Fitness Tracker:** Fitbit Alta HR
  - Step tracking and the Fitbit app for food logging
- **Bluetooth Scale:** FitIndex Bluetooth Scale
  - Logging weight and syncing to Fitbit app
- **The Freeze:** Isavera Ab Ice Wrap and Isavera Thigh Ice Wraps
- **The Freeze Massage:** OPOVE M3 Pro Percussion Massager

THE PROCESS

Every morning after waking up, I weighed myself before drinking or eating anything. This left me with a lot of useful data and weight charts in the Fitbit app. When I tracked my weight loss progress over the course of six months, what I saw was a straight, downward trending line.

Can you lose more than 35 pounds over the course of six months using this plan? Of course. If you have a lot of weight to drop, you will probably lose more.

In my experience, the fat I had to lose after my first 15 pounds was the type of stubborn fat that never goes away. Once you reach that point (which you will), the temptation to quit starts popping up. This is where the fat-freezing protocol helps keep you motivated. We'll also talk about overcoming mental hurdles soon in Part III: *Mindset and Muscle*.

STEPS

I aimed to walk at least ten thousand steps a day. I sometimes logged over ten thousand steps if I got distracted while listening to an audiobook or watching HBO on the treadmill.

During this case study, I hit ten thousand steps almost every day. On average, I hit between seventy thousand and eighty-five thousand steps a week. A light home treadmill will become your best friend to hit your step goals, but going for walks outside is an easy way to rack up steps without even thinking about it.

THE FREEZING PROCESS

My abs and thighs had the most fat to lose, so I targeted those areas to speed up fat loss. I used the Isavera ab wrap or the Isavera thigh wraps two to three times per week for an hour each session. This meant that sometimes I only froze my abs twice a week and my legs once a week or vice versa. Your goal should be to get two to three sessions per week total, regardless of the area. This way, you build a routine and ensure consistent fat freezing.

You can do more than three sessions a week if you're motivated. Doing more than three helps, but I recommend starting slow, so you can stay consistent. Consistency matters more than intensity when it comes to weight loss. There were sessions where I used both the ab and leg wraps simultaneously. You can do this to target a wider area of fat in your sessions. I recommend trying this approach if you have more than one version of the Isavera wraps.

My sessions were usually toward the end of the day, around 7:00 or 8:00 p.m. After I lost 25 pounds, I started using ice wraps less frequently. Toward month four, I used them only once or twice a week, but I continued to see good results.

Each time I used ice wraps, I made sure they were fully frozen. This is more important than you think;

you don't want to waste sessions with half-frozen ice packs.

I had a DEXA body fat scan performed around month six and found I had achieved 9 percent body fat. DEXA scans use a type of x-ray machine that provides very precise body fat measurements. Once I hit 9 percent body fat, I was actually motivated to start using the ice wraps more frequently and pushed to get fully chiseled abs once and for all.

MASSAGING POST FREEZE

The massager tools that come with the Isavera ice wraps worked well, but I started using a percussion massager around month four.

I felt that the percussion massager made a difference in my progress and brought much more circulation to the area. Not only was it good for use after a fat-freezing session, but it also worked wonders on sore muscles. The percussion massager is helpful, but it isn't necessary for you to see great results using the Isavera ice wraps.

THE FITBIT WEIGHT CHARTS

The Fitbit app aggregates your weekly average weight after each week is over. Even if your daily weight is up and down, you can compare your weekly averages and will likely notice a downward trend. I lost, on average, 1 to 2 pounds a week following the *Ice Sculpture Diet*.

At certain points during the six months, my weight stayed virtually the same across two weeks. That's what I call standing in the land of plateaus, but I stuck with tracking, getting steps, and freezing. Inevitably, I broke through this plateau a few weeks later. Stick with the plan during these times, and it will work for you.

THE FOOD LOG

I ate right at my BMR calorie level for almost the entire weight-loss cycle. Once or twice, I crossed over 2,000 calories a day by accident. This happened after eating out at a restaurant, only to realize that the food had more calories than I estimated once I logged it.

To avoid eating over my BMR, I learned to log my

food before eating it. On days where I went over 2,000 calories, I tried to walk twelve thousand or more steps to burn extra. Remember that two thousand steps is about 1 mile, which comes out to between 50–100 calories burned, depending on your body size.

What's most important here is not your daily calories but average weekly calories. You may eat over your BMR on some days, but you can make up for it by being more conscious the rest of the week and keeping your average weekly calories on track. If you're exercising along with tracking steps, you can eat over your BMR, as long as you're reasonable when logging calories burned for the additional exercise. The goal is to have a caloric deficit each day. That's how you lose weight.

With all the data you'll have in your Fitbit or MyFitnessPal app, it's easy to see how weight loss is a science. All of the numbers get logged just about daily, many of them automatically (steps, weight, calories burned). When you review your numbers and see progress each week, you'll be motivated to keep moving forward.

THE SUPPLEMENTS

During this six-month period, I took several supplements to keep my health in check. The only specific weight-loss supplement I took daily was 500 mg of green tea extract, which has many other benefits aside from slightly increasing metabolism.

Here's a list of some other supplements I took consistently:

- High EPA/DHA fish oil
- Multivitamin
- Vitamin D
- Curcumin Extract
- Purple Wraath BCAA while fasting (amino acids to maintain muscle mass)

All of these helped me achieve a healthy nutrient intake while watching what I ate, but they aren't all necessary for success. I recommend a multivitamin at the very least, and research the remaining supplements to see if they are right for you.

THINGS I WOULD DO DIFFERENTLY IF I STARTED OVER

There are a couple of things I'd do differently if I started the *Ice Sculpture Diet* routine over again.

When I started using the ice wrap protocol, I didn't take the initial waist, arm, and thigh measurements using the measuring tape that comes with the Isa-vera wraps. I had some mental blocks, thinking that measurements didn't matter if I could see the difference in the mirror anyway.

I regret not taking those measurements because I lost a ton of weight, and my waist and thighs shrunk considerably. I wish I had logged measurements like I logged everything else because then I'd have even more evidence and data to share with you.

So, when you're starting the *Ice Sculpture Diet*, use a tape measure to take your waist, hip, thigh, and arm measurements. FitIndex (the brand of Bluetooth scale I use) also makes a Bluetooth body tape measure to make logging your measurements in their app easier. You will thank yourself for taking measurements later, especially on the days when the scale isn't moving. On those days, you can look at your measurements and see the progress you're making. Measurements also help you see what the ice wraps are doing for you since ice wraps target subcutaneous fat specifically.

Another thing I'd do differently is buy more foods with barcodes. I switched to doing this around month four, and it made logging food a lot easier.

The trickiest thing you'll bump into with food tracking is logging complex meals. You'll likely underestimate the calories in these meals. I recommend purchasing food with barcodes and easy serving sizes like "1 cup" or "10 pita chips" so that you can log exactly what you're eating. Doing this, you can easily scan the barcode using your food-logging app's barcode scanner feature to keep track.

One more thing: pay attention to the number of servings listed on food packages. You may accidentally consume more calories than intended by not looking at the number of servings per container. One example of serving size surprise for me was finding out that many cans of tuna have two servings in them. While the cans are small, a serving of tuna is around 50 calories. If you missed the servings per container on the label, you'd think a can of tuna is 50 calories per can instead of 100 calories. Paying close attention here will help avoid weight loss confusion later.

WRAPPING UP

There will be times when the scale won't move at all—sometimes for a couple of weeks at a time. I found this frustrating even when I was expecting it. I learned that you have to keep pushing through these moments knowing that what you're following is a proven plan.

The beauty of this program is that *The Foundation* sets you up for success. Then, *The Freeze* pushes you past the doubts. You have to lose at least some fat when you're freezing on top of dieting, so increase your ice wrap frequency when you inevitably hit a plateau.

Keep your chin up during these times. If you want to do more, add some extra steps throughout the day, and make sure what you're eating is exactly what you're logging. You can also decrease your daily food intake by 100 calories until you see the scale move. In doing all this, you will make it to the finish line, especially with the help of Part III—*Mindset and Muscle*—coming up.

You may notice that weight comes off quicker at the beginning of your diet. This is common with all diets, as your body starts to get rid of some excess water weight. Your metabolism is also generally higher at the beginning of your diet. Celebrate this early weight loss, but don't use weight loss progress as an excuse to cheat.

Set your goal weight, set a date for it, calculate how many weeks you need and at what calorie level you should eat, and keep moving toward that point until you're there.

You will battle yourself during this process. Sometimes your mind won't *let* you lose weight because you don't believe you should be at that new weight level or because you believe your goal is impossible. You'll learn to work through those obstacles in the next part of this book.

In the upcoming chapters, I'm going to present a way of welcoming your new weight loss into your life and overcoming the mental blocks that prevent so many people from achieving their ideal weight. I'm also going to show you how to build this diet into a routine to make achieving your weight loss effortless. Finally, I'll show you how to add some muscle mass after you lose weight.

You've made it this far, so turn the page and get ready to overcome your greatest obstacle: your mind.

PART III

MINDSET AND MUSCLE

CHAPTER 8

WELCOMING A NEW YOU

Read the following sentence and fill in the blank with the first thought that pops into your mind:

I can lose 20 pounds over the next six months.

First thought (did you catch it?): _____

Notice the message that pops into your head. Watch the beliefs that start to bubble up when you read that sentence. If you thought something along the lines of, *No way, I can't do that*, then you're holding a limiting belief that may stop you from achieving your weight-loss goal.

This chapter is about the beliefs that appear in our minds when we start to lose weight and how to overcome them. These beliefs are real, and they will get in the way. Your subconscious mind can block your path if it thinks you are achieving something you don't believe you deserve. I wrote this chapter to protect you from this dilemma.

There's great work to be done here and a lot to learn about ourselves, so let's get started.

THE COMMON BELIEFS THAT SHOW UP

One of my favorite books is called *The Big Leap* by Gay Hendricks. This book discusses an idea called the Upper Limit problem." The idea behind the upper limit problem is that all people have an upper limit for what they believe is achievable in their lives. When you begin to get close to your limit, you subconsciously sabotage yourself and move back down to a level where you again feel comfortable.

When I read *The Big Leap* years ago, it was an awakening for me. I realized its message could be applied to so many different areas of my life, including weight loss.

So, how does the upper limit problem connect to the *Ice Sculpture Diet*? Well, as you start to see your weight dropping on the scale, your mind might pop out a few messages like the following:

- I'm losing too much weight! I should stop
- I've lost enough weight already; I should start eating more
- I deserve ice cream after all this effort
- I did good enough; no need to go any further
- I was just being hard on myself; it's okay to stop now
- I can't believe the scale isn't moving anymore; I guess I won't achieve my goal; I'll just call it quits here.
- Maybe I wasn't meant to be lean and fit; maybe that's for other people; it's not my destiny

Do any of these messages sound familiar? These are common beliefs people have while going through any diet. If you're familiar with one or more of these, it's probably because your mind repeats them constantly.

Take a moment to think about this:

What if you could achieve the ideal weight you set out to achieve?

You've already seen that weight loss can be calculated using easy math. It's a science. You can depend on the *Ice Sculpture Diet* working just like you can count on a ball coming down when you throw it in the air. The only two things stopping you from getting to where you want to be is an understanding of weight loss, which you have, and the mindset and willpower to achieve it. If you follow the steps outlined in this book—food logging, hitting ten thousand steps, and wearing ice wraps two to three times a week—you will reach your goal. Knowing this should help improve your willpower as well.

It sounds achievable when you look at it as a process, doesn't it? And that's because it is achievable. To move forward in our journey, we must overcome what the voice in our head tells us when we start losing weight.

We do that by writing a new story.

WRITING A NEW STORY

When you step on the scale and hear one of the thoughts listed above, say to yourself, *Anthony told me this message was going to pop into my head. Since I knew it was going to happen, I can accept it as part of the process, let it go, and continue going forward. No hurt feelings, no discouragement. It's all a part of the process.*

You can get past these beliefs by realizing and accepting that they are a part of you, and they are going to come. So, when they do appear, write a new story. Recognize that the thought is there, make a statement to counter it, let it go, and keep moving. That's all there is to it.

MOVING FORWARD TO THE NEW YOU

As you start to lose weight, you're going to notice a few things happening. You're going to notice changes in parts of your body that you never paid attention to before.

For example, I never realized how bony my hips were until I lost the first 20 pounds. As I started losing weight, I remember thinking, *What if I*

bump into something now? It's really going to hurt!
Isn't that silly? Who cares! But that silly message
had the potential to halt my progress. I could have
used it as an excuse to stop, and people do this all
the time, but I acknowledged the thought as an
expected message during this process and kept on
with the plan.

Many people use loose skin as an excuse to stop. If
you're experiencing loose skin, that's a great sign
that you're making progress. If you're worried about
this, some people advocate using creams for loose
skin. I have had a lot of success by simply losing
more weight and watching the skin slowly shrink
away. Adding some muscle mass helps too (see the
final chapter for this).

Remember that overcoming your weight-loss
beliefs takes time, but don't stop yourself just
because you aren't there yet. Turn the beliefs that
come up into motivation to keep pushing forward.
You can see these thoughts appearing and realize
they're a sign you're making progress. You can
worry about the excuses after you hit your goal.

ALLOWING YOUR NEW SELF-IMAGE TO EMERGE

Bob Proctor, a famous motivational speaker, helped me see the importance of cultivating a healthy self-image. If you want to more easily achieve your weight goals, you need to reshape the way you envision and talk about yourself.

When I started designing the *Ice Sculpture Diet*, I was around 190 pounds. As I approached 165 pounds, I kept having this nagging thought that I was becoming too small. I had been into bodybuilding since high school, and I always wanted to be as big and muscular as possible.

Was 165 pounds really the weight of a small, fragile guy? No! Some of the greatest boxers in the world are at that weight level. Floyd Mayweather only weighs 150 pounds, and nobody wants to mess with him. So, why was this idea in my head? I have no clue, but I realized it was stopping me from achieving my goal.

From that point on, I rewrote the script in my mind and changed my self-image. I changed the way I saw myself. I imagined that I was meant to be 165 pounds. I saw that my 190-pound self was actually a deviation from my ideal self. It was a result of drinking and eating too much back in my college days. I am much healthier at 165 pounds than I ever was at 190 pounds.

I replaced that old self-image and blasted past the 165-pound mark. As I'm writing this, I am now 155 pounds and have less than 9 percent body fat.

GOAL SETTING AND REFRAMING

How much do you weigh now? Where do you want to be in the next three to six months?

Imagine yourself there for a moment.

What thoughts pop into your head when you think about reaching that weight?

Grab a piece of paper and write those thoughts down or open the note app on your phone and type them in.

Then, write a reframe for every message you see.

Example: *I've tried to hit __ pounds before and failed.*

Reframe: *I have a system now and know weight loss is a science. I will reach my target ___-pound goal by following this process starting today.*

Through reframing, you can tackle the beliefs that block your way. By doing this, you allow yourself to accept a new self-image that will guide you through to the end. Read the thoughts you wrote down, reframe them, and let them go. You'll feel much freer once you do.

MINDSET SUMMARY

In this chapter, we talked about your mind and how it can prevent you from succeeding. We explored your beliefs, you looked at your story, and you've worked on and thought about your new self-image. You're even prepared to reframe your limiting beliefs as they pop up so that you can easily achieve your target weight.

With an understanding of how your mind affects you, it's time to talk about how you can automate your way past these mental obstacles. In the next chapter, we'll focus on creating routines to make reaching your goals effortless. Turn the page now

to learn how to build the *Ice Sculpture Diet* into a
habit with ease.

CHAPTER 9

ROUTINES FOR LONG-TERM WEIGHT LOSS

Remember that friend from Chapter 1? The guy or gal who'd tried every other diet and exercise plan out there but always seemed to look the same a few months later? If they chose just one of those plans, built habits around it, and stuck with it—they'd probably see a lot more success.

In this chapter, we'll talk about how to build the *Ice Sculpture Diet* into a mental routine, so you can stay on track and easily hit your goals. By the end, you'll have a set of habits that allow you to turn your weight loss on autopilot. I'll also be sharing a one-page template for the program to motivate you during your first few weeks on the diet.

WHY DO PEOPLE YO-YO?

Dieters often fall into the trap of "yo-yoing," where they lose and regain the same weight back. One reason this happens is that they don't stick with a plan long enough to adapt to a long-term, healthy lifestyle. They may try one thing, try another thing, and binge on pizza for a few weeks before reevaluating their diet plan.

Another reason people yo-yo is because they hold beliefs about themselves and about weight loss that cause them to bounce right back to a comfortable weight level for them. If you read and absorbed the last chapter, you're already way ahead of the pack on this one. If you're still concerned about these thoughts, go back and read the last chapter to overcome this.

The final reason people yo-yo is that they never created a routine to overcome resistance. A routine is the key ingredient for keeping weight off for the long-term. With a routine, you build the new you day by day. Your progress becomes automatic, and your goals become easily attainable.

WHY HABITS AND ROUTINES WORK

Any top athlete or top performer has a routine for their work. They practice something every day, repeating the key steps over and over. If they miss a day, they bounce back. Why do they bounce back so quickly? Because the habitual practice makes coming back automatic and effortless.

Building a routine takes a little bit of work up front, but all top performers know that some upfront effort pays off long term. Soon enough, practice becomes part of their regular life. They don't have to decide when and where to focus on their craft.

When you build a daily practice into your life, your mind adjusts. Routines work because they change you. After some time, you won't need to put in so much effort since your practice will become a normal part of life that you enjoy.

INTENSITY VS. CONSISTENCY

When I was younger and visited the gym with my friends in high school, we had one mission: to get huge. We started off by bench pressing every day, with terrible form, and working out all the wrong muscle groups to try to get that Brad Pitt *Fight Club* look. No more than three weeks after starting, our bodies were destroyed. I was pretty sure I had a torn rotator cuff, and I almost quit working out right then and there.

Thankfully, that setback didn't stop us forever. We picked ourselves back up and took it at a slower and steadier pace. We created a routine to work out, rather than an all-out extreme session on random days of the week.

Several years after developing a routine, it dawned on me that the issue back then wasn't the exercises that we were doing; it was that we went in like a loaded rocket ship and used up all of our fuel. We started off way too intense, and we couldn't sustain that pace.

The secret here is that consistency beats out intensity almost every time, especially if you're aiming to have long-term results.

Someone who works out or follows a simple diet plan every week for a year is going to have significantly better results (and longer-term results) than someone who works out randomly or diets for a few months, only to jump back into their old habits.

The consistency of a routine will lead to incremental improvements in your body each week. These incremental improvements accumulate over time, and you'll look amazing soon enough.

GUIDELINES FOR THE ICE SCULPTURE DIET ROUTINE

Here are some bullet points to guide you when setting up a routine for the *Ice Sculpture Diet*:

- Log all meals and any snacks *before* eating the food in your food-tracking app *daily*.
- Review your weekly average calories every Saturday to make sure the numbers are in line with your target BMR. You can do this in the Fitbit app or by adding up the last seven days of your calorie intake and dividing that number by seven.
- Pick one to three days a week, at the same hour each day, to use ice wraps on your target areas.

Picking the same hour each day helps turn it into a habit.

- If hitting ten thousand steps a day is a challenge, pick a specific hour of the day to go for a brisk walk. Walk extra on the weekends or days when you have more free time. Aim for your total weekly steps to be seventy thousand or more.

By following a routine, you make the *Ice Sculpture Diet* an everyday thing in your mind. This plan is not a *follow it on some days and not others* routine. Make it a daily practice, and it will become natural after the first two weeks. Wake up each morning and say to yourself, "I am following my plan today, and I am succeeding at it." If you struggle with willpower, push to keep yourself motivated for at least the first two to three weeks.

Finally, make your weight loss goal a part of your new identity. Regularly look in the mirror and thank yourself for putting in the effort to achieve your goal. Congratulate yourself for making it this far into the book. Find simple ways to celebrate the progress you're making, so you have wins to look back on as you progress.

HOW LONG DOES IT TAKE TO BUILD A HABIT?

Research on habit building varies, but the consensus is that it takes between twenty-one and sixty days to fully build a habit into your subconscious mind. Now, does that mean the first twenty-one days are going to be painful? Not at all. You're making a change, and change can be fun.

That said, the first two weeks of a routine are the most important. You need to keep this routine going every day so that your mind adapts to the changes. As you move into the habit, you will learn new things about yourself and your body. By seeing the data in your apps, you're going to find yourself curious to learn more and see continued progress. Soon, after two weeks or so, you'll be in your routine.

Once you're following the plan regularly, you can more easily bounce back from an off day here and there because your routine will kick back into place. Your mind has created guardrails around your new lifestyle, and it will help you stick to this plan.

A TEMPLATE FOR THE *ICE SCULPTURE DIET*

Set aside some time to write down your routine. Start to imagine the location where you will sit during your ice wrap routine, the consistent time period you will allot to getting your steps in, and the grocery shopping you will do to find healthy foods that fit within your BMR threshold.

To help you with your routine planning, I've included a one-page template for the *Ice Sculpture Diet* routine on the next page. Use this to make your routine fun. When you're first starting, check it every day to see if you can get the highest score. Work with this template to stay motivated until you don't need it anymore.

You can download a PDF version of this template to print by visiting: icesculpturediet.com/template.

THE ICE SCULPTURE DIET TEMPLATE

INSTRUCTIONS:

- Take a photo or print this template out. Each template covers five weeks on the plan.
- On days that you freeze, put a letter **F** in the box for that day of the week. Aim for two to three freeze sessions per week.
- On days that you walked ten thousand steps, put a letter **W** in that box. Your goal should be to have a W in every box at the end of the week.
- On days where you ate close to your BMR, put a letter **B** in that box. If you ate above your BMR but exercised to make up for it, you can write a **B** in the box.

WEEK	S	M	T	W	T	F	S	TOTAL
1								
2								
3								
4								
5								

F = 2.5 points (7.5 max) | B = 2 points | W = 1.5 points

EACH WEEK—ADD UP YOUR SCORE:

- **0-10:** Needs work
- **11-20:** Okay—almost there
- **21-31:** You will achieve your goal
- **32:** Rock star! Six-pack status

ICE SCULPTURE DIET APPROVED PRODUCTS:
ICESCULPTUREDIET.COM/RECS

- Isavera Abdominal Fat-Freezing Belt
- Fitbit Fitness Tracker
- FitIndex Bluetooth Scale
- Jarrow Green Tea Extract (Natural Fat Burner)

CHAPTER 10

BONUS: BUILDING MUSCLE AFTER WEIGHT LOSS

You've walked through *The Foundation* for fat loss, *The Freeze* for overcoming plateaus, and the first two chapters of *Mindset and Muscle* to move past your subconscious weight-loss blocks. What's left? It's time to build some muscle.

As you start losing weight, you may find yourself curious about getting more active and toning your muscles. People often have even more motivation to do this if they notice some flabbiness (loose skin) on their arms, thighs, stomach, or even chest after a successful diet.

One of the quickest ways to get a nice lean look after dieting is to begin strength training, so you can add lean muscle mass where you lost fat. We'll talk about how to do that in this chapter, so you can achieve your ideal look.

If you're not interested in gaining muscle now, that's fine. Reaching your weight-loss goal was your mission, and if you accomplished that goal, congratulations are in order.

Consider this chapter a bonus. You can always come back to it if you're curious about building muscle in the future. There are a lot of benefits that come with exercising, and we'll talk about that here as well.

MUSCLE GROWTH

I'm a certified personal trainer and have been working out for around fifteen years now. In this chapter, I'm going to show you the common issues people face when trying to gain muscle. I'm also going to show you how to overcome those traps and outline a few key exercises for each body part to help get you started off strong.

COMMON PITFALLS WHEN GAINING MUSCLE MASS

Many new exercisers don't reach their muscle-mass goals for two main reasons.

First: they lack consistency.

You learned how important routines were in the last chapter. The key to proper muscle growth is to set a timeline and schedule. Just as habits apply with weight loss, they apply with gaining muscle as well.

To see progress from weightlifting, I recommend training three to four times a week.

You'll need to focus on specific strength exercises for each muscle group to see progress. You will learn the exercises I love and recommend in this chapter. With a consistent schedule for these exercises, you can start to see results in as little as a month.

EATING ENOUGH FOOD FOR MUSCLE RECOVERY

The second reason people have trouble building muscle mass is their food intake. You have to eat more protein and maintain a certain level of calories to gain muscle. When you want to gain muscle mass and tone your body, you should plan to eat a little bit over your BMR.

I am not saying you should eat whatever you want and call it a "bulk" cycle (like some people do). That will only reverse the progress you've made on the *Ice Sculpture Diet* so far and leave you with additional fat. Instead, the extra calories should come mostly from protein and fiber-filled vegetables. You have to eat more protein when strength training because protein is used for muscle repair. Aim to consume 0.5 to 1 gram of protein per pound of body weight each day. This way, your body will have enough amino acids (broken-down protein) for muscle recovery.

HOW MUSCLE GROWTH WORKS

So, how do you gain lean mass? Here's how it works: strength training causes small tears in your muscle fibers. When your body repairs these tears, it adds mass to the muscle groups being repaired. Over time, you begin to accumulate a lot of additional mass by performing steady weightlifting sessions.

It will be easier to gain muscle mass when you're

finished dieting. When you're on a diet and in a caloric deficit, you likely won't have enough calories to properly fuel your muscle growth. Your body won't be focusing on muscle repair if you're not providing it enough nutrients to repair your muscles after a workout. Taking amino acid supplements can help, but eating more is the better option.

You can strength train while dieting, but the mass gains will be limited until you start eating more. Still, I love working out, even if I am dieting, because of the way it makes me feel. Do what feels right for you and make sure you are sticking to a plan.

THE BENEFITS OF HAVING MUSCLE

Strength training has a lot of benefits beyond just building muscle mass. I have a saying that I'd like you to internalize: "Life is better with more muscle." Now, there are definitely some people that go overboard with this and injure themselves in a never-ending pursuit of mass. In general, though, there are a ton of great benefits that come with adding a few additional pounds of muscle to your body.

For one thing, muscle mass burns more calories

than fat does. In other words, having more muscle mass increases your BMR. If you're able to pack on a decent amount of muscle, say 10 or more pounds, your body will not only look more toned, but you'll be burning off more calories throughout the day.

Strength training has also been shown to increase bone density. This is especially important as you get older. Studies show that people who strength train are less likely to have issues with osteoporosis and bone fractures. This makes sense; having denser bones makes them generally less likely to break.

Strength training also releases endorphins in your brain. These are the chemicals that give you that happy feeling after a nice workout. This explains why people can get addicted to working out (myself included). It's because working out makes you feel great. The same applies to the "runner's high" that marathon runners experience. Studies have also shown that exercise improves blood oxygen levels in the brain for several hours after you work out. This is great for brain health and recovery.

One last and obvious benefit: the more muscle mass you have, generally the more strength you possess. You can carry heavier things, do a pull-up or push-up easily, and do tasks around the house with ease.

Now that you've learned about some of the benefits of gaining muscle, it's time to learn a few excellent exercises to get you started.

What follows are the exercises I recommend for each muscle group and a description of how to perform each exercise. For this section, if you are unsure how to perform any exercise properly, I recommend you watch a few YouTube videos on it. My descriptions will help, but watching videos will make it easier for you. This will help ensure your exercise form is correct and prevents injuries. Like with any change in diet, you should consult your doctor before making changes to your current exercise routine (be safe!).

ICE SCULPTURE DIET ARM EXERCISES

Your arms have several distinct muscle groups, but we'll focus on growing the biceps and triceps.

Many weightlifters focus only on their biceps for

the peak, but the size of your arms is heavily influenced by the size of your triceps. If you want big arms, you have to work out your triceps. Trust me on this one.

BICEP EXERCISES

The two main exercises we'll be doing for biceps are the **bicep curl** and the **hammer curl**.

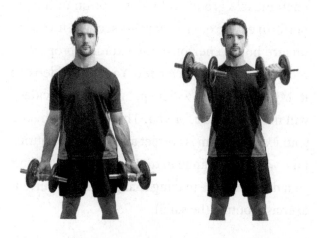

The regular bicep curl is a great way to build the peak in your bicep, so you have that rounded look even when your muscle is unflexed. When doing the bicep curl, keep your upper arm (above the elbow) straight in line with your body while curling the weight up toward your shoulder. Do not swing the weight as you bring it up, as this takes the tension off the bicep muscle. Focus on making it a smooth and controlled motion when raising the weight up.

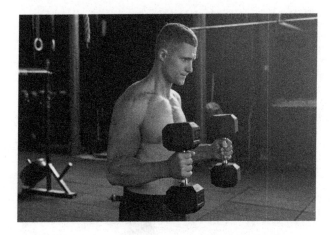

The hammer curl is a variation of the bicep curl, following the same up and down motion. The difference with the hammer curl is that you rotate your wrists, so you hold the dumbbells in a vertical position instead of a horizontal position. The hammer curl places more emphasis on the long head of the bicep muscle, giving your arm a nice overall pop and adding additional mass.

Make sure, again, to keep your arm straight in line with your body when performing both bicep curls and hammer curls. This keeps most of the tension on your biceps instead of other muscle groups like the back or legs (for folks that like to push off the ground while curling).

TRICEPS EXERCISES

Just like for biceps, there are two main exercises we'll focus on for developing our triceps. The first exercise is the **overhead triceps extension**, and the second exercise is the pulley or bent over dumbbell **triceps kickback**.

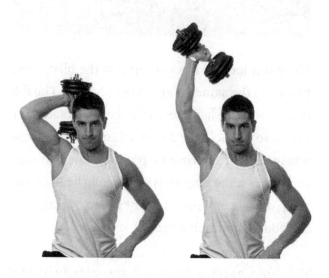

Overhead triceps extensions involve lifting a single dumbbell with two hands or two dumbbells (one in each hand) over your head and slowly lowering the weight behind your head. From behind your head, use your triceps to lift the weight back overhead to the starting position. Keep your elbows pointing straight toward the ceiling so that you maintain good form and keep the tension hitting directly on your triceps (the back of your arms).

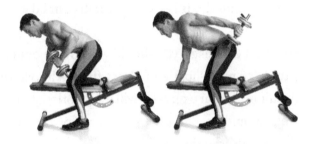

Triceps kickbacks can be done using a cable pulley adjusted to the height of your shoulders when bending forward at a 45-degree angle. This exercise can also be done with dumbbells while bending over at the same 45-degree angle.

The goal of this exercise is to start with the elbow and upper arm in line with your body. Straighten your arm, pivoting off your elbow, using your triceps to move the weight upwards and back. Your upper body should remain bent forward at a 45-degree angle from your waist, with your feet firmly planted, to hit the triceps more directly. This exercise is great for targeting the triceps and, when done consistently, will add a lot of mass to the backs of your arms.

ICE SCULPTURE DIET CHEST EXERCISES

Building your chest, or your pectorals, and front shoulder muscles is key to an overall defined look.

For chest exercises, you should go with the **bench press** (or push-ups) and **chest flies**. Almost all pushing-motion exercises will also work out your front shoulders, so we won't be focusing on shoulder exercises in this section.

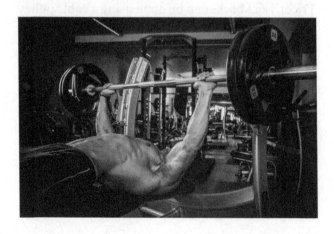

The bench press is a very popular exercise and simple to perform once you have the motion figured out. Lay flat on a weight bench and push the barbell up off the rack. You should use your chest, triceps, and front shoulders for this movement. Lower the weight down to have it touch your chest lightly and push, focusing on your chest, to bring it back to the starting position.

Form is important for the bench press. Incorrect motions can leave you with an injured rotator cuff due to putting too much pressure on the shoulders instead of the pectorals. The key to this exercise is making sure your elbows are at roughly a 45-degree angle from your sides. You do not want your elbows to be flailed out in line with your shoulders. Flailing your elbows is what puts excess pressure on your shoulders. Keep your elbows tucked in, closer to the sides of your body, but with a little space so that you feel the muscle tension primarily on your chest.

Do bench presses for three to five sets of eight to ten repetitions. You want the last repetition to be hard but not so hard that you get stuck with the weight on your chest.

The same bench press form principles also apply for push-ups. Keep your back straight when doing pushups, no arching, and do as many push-ups as you can for three to five sets. The bench press is the better option for gaining muscle mass, but you can definitely gain strength and some mass doing push-ups if you don't have access to a bench press setup. I recommend buying a Perfect Pushup to take some of the pressure off your wrists when doing push-ups.

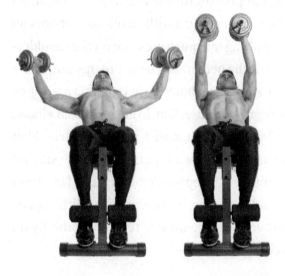

Chest flies focus on the outer ends of the pectoral muscles. You should do chest flies either lying down on a bench using dumbbells or using a chest-fly machine. If you use dumbbells, the motion is to lift the weights above your chest while laying down, slowly lowering the weights outwards toward your sides, and then bringing them back to the starting position above your chest.

The key for chest-fly form is to make sure your arms are straight with a slight bend in the elbow as you bring the weight down to your sides. This means adjusting the weight to a level where you can easily lower it down to your sides without overly bending your elbows. If you bend your elbows too much, it reduces the range of motion for the exercise. Start off with 5- or 10-pound dumbbells and see how that feels before increasing the weight. Three sets of five to ten repetitions should do the job.

ICE SCULPTURE DIET LEG EXERCISES

For legs, we'll focus on just the **squat**. The squat is the ultimate leg exercise and is considered a compound exercise, meaning that it works many different muscle groups at once. The squat and the deadlift are two of the best exercises for gaining muscle mass.

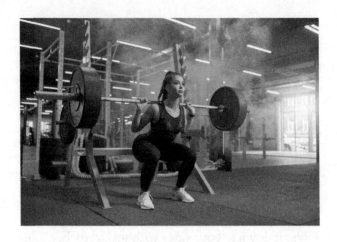

Place a barbell on your shoulders, slowly squat down toward the ground, then thrust yourself up into a standing position using mainly your hamstrings, glutes, hips, and quads. It sounds simple, but proper squat form is complex.

I recommend watching a few YouTube videos on squat form, in particular, to make sure you're doing it right. For starters: you want to make sure your back is not arching, your feet are roughly shoulder-width apart or a little wider, and that you don't lean forward when bringing the weight down. Balance and stance are very important for the squat because of the weight on your shoulders.

Do three to five sets of eight repetitions. You will be

sore after. When I tell you squats will build muscle mass, I mean it. You can add several pounds of muscle to your legs by doing squats alone. Squats also help build your core (abdominal region), which helps with overall stability and strength.

ICE SCULPTURE DIET BACK EXERCISES

There are two exercises I recommend for back muscles: **deadlifts** and **lat pull-downs**. Deadlifts are the king of all muscle-building exercises because, as a compound exercise, they hit so many different muscle groups simultaneously. These muscles include the lats, traps, quads, hamstrings, lower back muscles, biceps, your core, and even triceps.

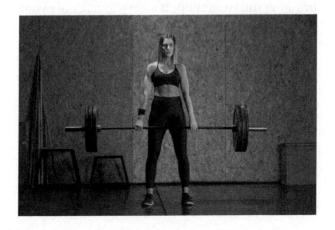

The basics of the deadlift are in the name. You're lifting a barbell off of the ground, up to about waist level, and then placing it back down to starting position—kind of like lifting a dead weight. Just because it sounds simple, though, doesn't mean it's easy.

Deadlift form, like squat form, is highly prone to error. This is one exercise where you should definitely watch a video to ensure proper form. Doing these incorrectly will cause back pain. I say this from personal experience. I went to the chiropractor several times before I realized my deadlift form was messing up my back.

Here are a few keys for form: You should focus on using your legs for the starting motion when bringing the weight up. It's easy to use only your back muscle with deadlifts, but the starting action should be similar to the upward motion of a squat. Once the bar is at the knee level, begin straightening out your back until you are standing tall with your body fully engaged. Avoid arching your back when you're starting off the deadlift motion.

If you performed only deadlifts one to two times a week for a few months, you would gain a lot of muscle in your back. If you want to target the V-shape look in your back muscles a little bit more, use the lat pull-down machine or do regular pull-ups (note: not a chin-up). Look for the lat pull-down machine at your local gym or invest in a doorway pull-up bar. Sometimes these pull-up bars have dip bar attachments, making them a good investment for strengthening your back, biceps, and triceps from home. I have one in my doorway and find it was an amazing investment for the price.

ICE SCULPTURE DIET AB EXERCISES

Finally, we come to our abs, where many new body-builders focus. I'm going to break some news here, but you don't have to work out your abs all that much. If you are strength training, especially if you're doing deadlifts, squatting, and bench pressing, then your core muscles are probably already in great shape.

Even people that don't work out at all—if they have low body fat—naturally have visible abs. Making your abs visible is more about diet and fat loss than building muscle mass in your abdominal region.

Following the *Ice Sculpture Diet* in its entirety should

help you lose weight and see your abs again, so get started now. Once you're on that path, you can add in **planks** and **crunches** to build some additional definition.

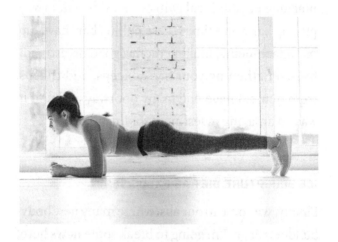

A plank seems childishly simple, but it is challenging to hold. Start in a push-up position and then move to rest your body weight on your forearms. Keep your back straight while doing this, tense your abs for additional focus, and hold this position for thirty seconds to one minute. Do this for two to three sets, up to five times a week. Planks hit your core muscles extremely well, and you will feel the burn quickly.

Besides planks, crunches are the go-to ab exercise

for most people. They're easy enough to do and can definitely add definition when performed on a consistent basis. When doing crunches, don't pull too forcefully on the back of your head with your hands. Your hands should lightly move with the back of your head while your abs do the work. Work your way to thirty to fifty crunches per set. If you get up to 100 crunches in a single set, your abs will really be developing. Start with however many crunches you can perform, though. Do this regularly, one or two times a week, and you will have all the ab muscle you need.

FREQUENCY FOR PERFORMING STRENGTH EXERCISES

When strength training, focus on hitting each muscle group and feeling the activation for each targeted muscle. There are many ways to organize workout routines, but I recommend going with a split routine. This means working two muscle groups a day, usually in these pairs:

- Chest and triceps
- Back and biceps
- Legs and shoulders

As with all things in the *Ice Sculpture Diet*, keep your routine simple. Aim to work out at least two times a week and work out muscle groups that you specifically want to grow. Once you get more comfortable working out, look to incorporate other exercises and pick it up to three or four sessions per week.

REST AND RECOVERY

Proper recovery is necessary for muscle growth. Recovery also includes sleep. In fact, your body does the majority of its muscle repair while you're sleeping.

The rule I follow for recovery is this: if you targeted a muscle today, don't work it out for two days. Smaller muscle groups (like biceps, triceps, and abs) can be worked out more frequently. Focus on making steady progress. You will find a rhythm to strength training, and the practice will add to the overall benefits you've experienced from the *Ice Sculpture Diet* so far.

A combination of weight loss and muscle growth will have you looking and feeling amazing in a few short months.

CONCLUSION

PUTTING IT ALL TOGETHER

Congratulations are in order. You've made it to the end of the *Ice Sculpture Diet*. By reaching this point, you've picked up everything you need to lose weight with ease.

You have your BMR calculated and memorized. You have a fitness tracker ready and hopefully started walking 10,000 steps a day. Your food-logging app has some data filled in, and your ice wraps are in the freezer, so you can start freezing fat. You've even put some thought into mental blocks and printed out the routine template to keep you moving.

All that is left now is to put this into motion and get started.

Before we part ways, let's solidify this process with a ten-step recap. You can come back to this whenever you need a reminder of the topics covered throughout the *Ice Sculpture Diet*.

SUMMARY AND CHAPTER INDEX

1. Understand and calculate your BMR (Chapter 2)
2. Begin logging your food (Chapter 3)
3. Eat enough healthy calories to be roughly at your BMR threshold (Chapters 3 and 4)
4. Walk 10,000 steps a day to create more of a caloric deficit (Chapter 3)
5. Leverage technology to keep your data synced; weigh yourself a few times a week, log your food, and track your steps (Chapter 4)
6. Use ice wraps around targeted areas, such as your waist and thighs, two to three times a week for continued fat reduction (Chapters 5 and 6)
7. Review the case study for tips to practice along the way (Chapter 7)
8. Prepare for the weight loss ahead with a new self-image and mindset (Chapter 8)

9. Build your routine to make this process automatic and easy to follow (Chapter 9)
10. If you're up for it, add some strength training exercises to replace lost fat with muscle and burn more calories (Chapter 10)

If you follow the ten steps outlined above for two to three months, you will see dramatic changes in the shape of your body. You'll be able to break through old plateaus and come out on the other side with confidence and a new view of what's possible.

STAY CONNECTED

I'm excited to have been a part of your weight-loss journey. I know how challenging it can be. I also know how great the rewards are when you reach the finish line.

Remember to track your progress and look back to stay motivated. Return to this book when you're having doubts. If you skipped some of the chapters mentioned in the outline above, go back and read them. While the ten-step process can seem simple, you'll be most successful when you understand the thinking behind each step. You can pass through many of the challenges ahead by getting back into the material, sharing it, and realizing you're following a system that works.

I hope you've enjoyed this journey. If this book has helped you, share the *Ice Sculpture Diet* with one friend who might enjoy it. If you have any questions or are looking for guidance, feel free to reach out to me. I'm excited to hear about your results following the plan.

You can find me by visiting my website: icesculp turediet.com. I read every message that comes in.

Stay cool and enjoy the progress ahead.

—ANTHONY D. GALLO

Made in the USA
Middletown, DE
12 May 2021

39534417R00099